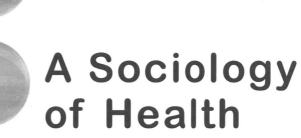

A Sociology of Health

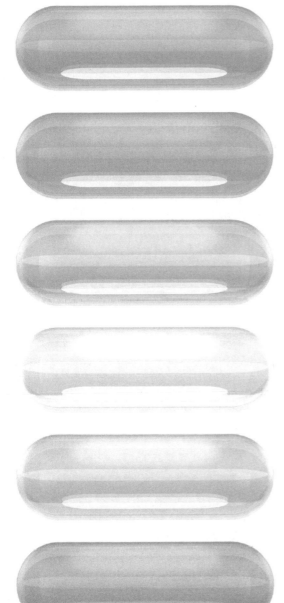

A Sociology of Health

Edited by
David Wainwright

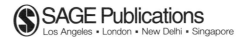

SAGE Publications
Los Angeles · London · New Delhi · Singapore

First published 2008

SAGE Publications Ltd
1 Oliver's Yard
55 City Road
London EC1Y 1SP

SAGE Publications Inc.
2455 Teller Road
Thousand Oaks, California 91320

SAGE Publications India Pvt Ltd
B 1/I 1 Mohan Cooperative Industrial Area
Mathura Road
New Delhi 110 044

SAGE Publications Asia-Pacific Pte Ltd
33 Pekin Street #02-01
Far East Square
Singapore 048763

Library of Congress Control Number: 2007929434

British Library Cataloguing in Publication data

A catalogue record for this book is available from the British Library

ISBN 978-1-4129-2157-2
ISBN 978-1-4129-2158-9 (pbk)

Typeset by C&M Digital Pvt Ltd, Chennai, India
Printed and bound in Great Britain by TJ International Ltd, Padstow, Cornwall
Printed on paper from sustainable resources

Contents

Preface

Social science may be confused, but its confusion should be exploited rather than bemoaned. It may be sick, but recognition of this fact can and should be taken as a call for diagnosis and perhaps even as a sign of coming health.

C. Wright Mills, *The Sociological Imagination*, 1959

While many medical sociologists are safely ensconced in departments of sociology and rarely teach students from outside their faculty, others are located in medical schools or other settings where they encounter a range of healthcare professionals both as students and research collaborators. First-year medical students, for example, are obliged to take a brief course introducing them to the social sciences as they are applied to medicine. The intention is to broaden the students' horizons beyond the realm of medical science and enable them to develop an awareness of the patient as a social being. Not surprisingly, many react against this imposition and would rather spend their scarce time on what they see as more clinically useful topics, such as neurology or anatomy. All too often what was intended to spark the sociological imagination of the healthcare professional, only serves as a vaccination against future contact with the discipline.

Teaching sociology to healthcare professionals can be a dispiriting occupation, but it does provide an insight into the uneasy relationship between the discipline and its subject matter. Qualitative researchers sometimes use the technique of 'informant validation' in which the results of the researcher's analysis are presented to those who participated in the study to see if they fit with the informants' own interpretations. The technique is of limited value because sociological analysis can reveal 'truths' about a group which are not apparent to its members, and to which they may take exception, but which are no less valid for that. But the antagonism between medical sociology and medical practitioners goes much deeper than that between analyst and analysed. It is not just that medical students take issue with some of the claims of sociology, but that they detect in it a hostile opposition to the principles of modern medicine and the implication that to practise medicine is an act of bad faith.

What the medical students pick up on are the claims that science should be given no primacy over other 'truth-claims', that medical knowledge is just a cloak for the exercise of professional power and that the putative achievements of medical practice are insignificant compared to the gains that could be made by addressing the social determinants of health. The spark for this book came not from those medical students who put up a spirited defence against such claims, but from the many others who acquiesced in them; from the growing number expressing the belief that homeopathy has an important role to play, or that the patient's diagnosis was every bit as valid as the doctor's. It occurred to me that this response was more in touch with the spirit of the times and reflected a broader malaise in the dominant medical institutions and elites.

For more than a generation medical sociology has defined itself in opposition to what James Le Fanu (1999) describes as the golden age of clinical science which emerged in the post-war period and which was characterised by commitment to the Enlightenment project of using science and reason to overcome the problems of humanity.[1] However, as Le Fanu has observed, this golden age was drawing to a close by the 1970s: medical science and the profession that practised it were increasingly challenged and questioned, not least by medical sociology. Of course, sociology should always question the established order and challenge orthodox ways of thinking about the world, and challenging the hubristic claims of modern medicine must have seemed radical and progressive at the time. However, in today's context there are new orthodoxies to be debunked, a new discourse of health to be critically explored.

The aim of this book is to apply a critical approach to the most pressing issues and controversies in the contemporary discourse of health. Central to our perspective is the belief that although the concepts, theories and methods of medical sociology (in its broadest sense) can aid our understanding of these issues and controversies, the discipline itself does not stand outside of its subject matter as an objective observer; but rather the social models which have emerged from medical sociology have themselves had a fundamental impact on the way in which health and illness are made sense of and understood in contemporary western societies. This influence has not always been progressive and much of what follows takes issue with many of the assumptions and claims of medical sociology; as such it is both an exposition and a critique of the discipline.

It is traditional for 'textbooks' to offer an even-handed *précis* of the canon; of course, perceptive students will always ask how the content of the canon was decided and what lies behind this claimed even-handedness. No such claims are made here. We have selected from medical sociology those concepts and theories which we believe have had most impact upon the new discourse of health, or which are of most value in understanding it. The contributors to the book are a diverse group, not all of whom would describe themselves as medical sociologists. They subscribe to no individual school of thought or uniform theoretical standpoint, but there are common threads running through their analyses. The achievements of medical science are recognised and valued, but there is also recognition that there is a social and psychological dimension to health and illness. Medical pluralism and epistemological relativism are eschewed, but there is recognition that knowledge is always socially situated and may (or may not) be distorted by vested interests. More importantly, there is a humanist orientation which emphasises the capacity for humans to make sense of the world around them and use reason to overcome the problems and difficulties they face. It is this humanist orientation and re-engagement with the Enlightenment project that gives the book its distinctive approach. As the chapters unfold it will become apparent that the new discourse of health is founded on a far gloomier interpretation of human potential.

The structure of the book

Chapter 1 provides a brief introduction to some of the key themes and contradictions that characterise the new discourse of health, before describing three social models of health and illness that have emerged from medical sociology and related disciplines such as epidemiology and social medicine. The three approaches are appraised in terms of their influence on the new discourse of health and in terms of their theoretical adequacy. The chapter closes with an outline sketch of what an alternative approach to the sociology of health and illness, grounded in critical realism and humanism, might look like. This new perspective is a work in progress rather than a firmly established and clearly defined paradigm. The remaining chapters provide examples of this approach in practice.

In **Chapter 2** Alan Buckingham asks why, after a century in which medical science made phenomenal progress in the fight against disease, we appear to have a heightened sense of anxiety about our health, which has led to ever greater regulation of perceived 'health risks' and 'unhealthy lifestyle choices'. Close analysis of the statistical evidence behind such health scares not only reveals that such claims are often based upon poor research or 'junk science', but that many of the statistical techniques employed by researchers exploring the social determinants of health and unhealthy lifestyles, even if applied with great rigour and precision, must inevitably give rise to a degree of anxiety which is disproportionate to the threat posed, for example, the calculation of relative rather than absolute risk ratios. The chapter concludes by considering the extent to which health statistics are both a cause and consequence of a broader culture of fear.

There is more to health and illness than the presence or absence of physical pathology. The western medical model is frequently criticised for its 'biological reductionism'; the failure to recognise the role of subjectivity and social relations in the aetiology, experience and outcome of illness and disease. Proponents of 'holistic medicine' have argued for greater understanding of the subjective aspects of suffering and a transcendence of mind–body dualism. In **Chapter 3** Stephen Bowler explores the mind–body problem, in the context of the humanist Enlightenment project. Where medical sociology has frequently viewed the objectification of the body as a limitation of the bio-medical gaze, Bowler argues that the capacity for science to master the objective reality of the body is central to the success of modern medicine. The current trend towards holistic and complementary medicine does not represent the emergence of more humane practice, so much as a loss of faith in human agency; a trajectory which leads away from science and medical progress.

Several chapters in this book refer to health scares or health risks, and the emergence of a heightened sense of mental and physical vulnerability. In **Chapter 4**, Adam Burgess asks what it is about contemporary western societies that provides such fertile ground in which the seeds of health risk can take root and flourish. Grounding his analysis in recent health scares, such as the putative link between the combined vaccination for Measles, Mumps and Rubella (MMR) and the onset of autism in childhood, and the equally spurious claims about health risks associated with the use of mobile phones, Burgess develops a multi-dimensional sociological framework which locates the preconditions for the risk society at the macro level of social development, the intermediate level of contextual factors, and the direct role of 'risk entrepreneurs' and other groups and institutions in promoting alarm.

Chapter 5 examines the influence that the three social models of health and illness have had on the broader discourse of health and illness through the New Public Health and the adoption of Patient Centred Practice in primary care. It is argued that the redefinition of health in terms of mental and social wellbeing has broadened the domain of healthcare policy and practice to include new areas of everyday life, while the identification of psycho-social stressors and lifestyle risk factors has given rise to a new sense of mental and physical vulnerability. At the same time, the role of the doctor as gatekeeper to the sick has been eroded by a shift from evidence of physical pathology as the basis of diagnosis, towards the subjective illness claims of the patient. These changes have contributed to an epidemic of medically unexplained illness behaviour and an expansion of the role of healthcare in the governance of everyday life.

The purpose of medicine is to ameliorate suffering, but the pursuit of this goal entails entering into a set of social relations that are embroiled in the exercise of power and control. Sociologists have conceptualised this contradiction through the category of medicalisation, and in **Chapter 6** Frank Furedi explores how this construct has been reformulated during its 40-year history. Emerging during the radical questioning of professional and institutional power of the late 1960s, medicalisation was initially coined as a challenge to the professional dominance of 'problems' such as madness, childbirth, and homosexuality. However, as Furedi's analysis reveals, the phenomenon of medicalisation has undergone a vault-face. Medicalisation no longer refers to the expanding power and influence of the medical profession, but to a broader cultural turn, in which diagnosis and therapy have become entangled in the validation of identity – ironically, the impetus for medicalisation no longer comes from the doctor but from the would-be patient.

Second-wave feminism made a significant contribution to the theory of medicalisation, and also provided its operational arm, in the form of the women's health movement of the 1970s; rejecting medicalised categories which asserted that women's subordinate role in society had a biological rather than political basis, and asserting the right for women to identify and address their own health needs. In **Chapter 7** Ellie Lee and Elizabeth Frayn document the retreat from this emancipatory standpoint, as contemporary feminists demand recognition of new medicalised categories such as Post-natal Depression or Pre-menstrual Syndrome, which imply that women *really are* slaves to their biology. The extent of this reversal is nowhere more apparent than in the rise of the men's health movement which is grounded in the critique of masculinity and encourages a more pusillanimous approach to the negotiation of health risks. The *feminization* of health is explored through a detailed case-study of the topical and controversial issue of cancer screening.

The uneasy relationship between medical science and medical sociology is woven deeply into the fabric of this book. In **Chapter 8** Tracey Brown explores this tension, placing the relativist challenge to medical knowledge in the broader context of the conflict between science and 'wilful superstition'. The rise of the evidence-based medicine movement is charted and the different strands of the backlash against it are discussed, from the feminist standpoint theory to complementary and alternative medicine. It is concluded that although medicine may have won the science wars, the victory is becoming increasingly pyrrhic, as leading scientific institutions and authorities retreat into defensive and conservative strategies.

In **Chapter 9** Mike Bury draws together many themes discussed earlier in the book and applies them to the latest policy initiatives relating to the National Health Service. Central to the analysis is the shifting relationship between the providers of health care and its recipients, variously constructed as: the public, consumers, partners, or expert patients. The medical profession have retained much of their social standing and trust, but in other respects they appear beleaguered; hemmed in by bureaucratic regulation and control, threatened by litigation, and obliged to cede authority to a range of competing interests. Rhetorically at least, the chief beneficiary of this apparent redistribution of power is the patient; empowered by new mechanisms of consumerism and choice, with their preferences and subjective beliefs buoyed to at least equal status with the expertise of the doctor. Yet all may not be as it seems and through a highly nuanced analysis the reality of this top down revolution in the doctor-patient relationship is revealed.

In the final chapter, **Chapter 10**, Vanessa Pupavac reveals how the tensions and uncertainties of western medicine are being exported to the developing world. Following the Second World War international health policy was linked to a broader project of economic and social modernisation, which saw the exportation of high-technology medicine to the towns and cities of the third world, coupled with ambitious public health programmes to eradicate smallpox and malaria. However, by the mid 1970s the modernisation agenda was faltering under criticisms that it was unaffordable, inappropriate and unsustainable. Modernisation gave way to the more modest goal of sustained development, and rather than attempting to equip the developing world with high-technology medicine international agencies shifted towards meeting basic health needs among the rural poor through deprofessionalised initiatives which often embraced traditional healing and environmentalist concerns. Earlier chapters describe the way in which the focus of health policy in the affluent West has shifted from the treatment of disease towards a broader pursuit of 'healthy lifestyles' and 'psycho-social wellbeing'; Pupavac's analysis reveals the extent to which this therapeutic model is being adopted by international aid and development agencies as a means of ameliorating the 'trauma' of poverty and hardship, but failing to address the core problems of uneven and unequal development.

Conclusion

Illness is not easy terrain for humanists; it is where we encounter our limitations. Ultimately physiology extinguishes human consciousness – death is the end of all our projects and aspirations. But it is also the place where we transcend at least some of these limitations in a uniquely human way. Animals do not make sense of their symptoms, they do not derive theories of aetiology, they have no system of diagnostic categories, and they have developed no curative treatments for their afflictions beyond the most basic adaptive responses. Humans do all of these things, not alone, but through social relations, lay and professional networks, and the production of knowledge. The profoundly social character of illness and medicine means that health can never be absolutely reduced to biological science. The sociological imagination has an important role to play in revealing the ways in which social relations influence how we make sense of our ailments and find ways of overcoming them. In the past the relationship between medical sociology and medical science has often been an antagonistic one. Social models of health have often been presented as a superior alternative to bio-medicine, and the Enlightenment claim that social progress results from the application of science to the natural world has been dismissed by some sociologists as a cloak for tyranny. Our purpose in writing this introductory text is to posit a very different relationship between medical sociology and its subject matter. A critical humanist approach to medical sociology is one which recognises the contribution that modern medicine can make to social progress and which uses the concepts and methods of sociological inquiry to reveal and understand the social and cultural obstacles to the realisation of that potential.

David Wainwright, Bath, April 2007.

References

1 Le Fanu, J. (1999) *The Rise and Fall of Modern Medicine*. London: Little Brown & Co.

Acknowledgements

I would like to thank everyone who has contributed to the production of this book. My co-authors have responded promptly and with good grace to requests for drafts and redrafts. The anonymous reviewers provided many helpful suggestions for improving the content and format of the book. The staff at SAGE have been supportive and helpful throughout, particularly Zoë Elliott-Fawcett and Anna Luker.

Epigraphs

The editor would like to thank the copyright holders for permission to reproduce the following quotations:

Foreword epigraph:
Wright Mills (1963). Reproduced with permission of Oxford University Press, Inc.

Chapter 1 epigraph:
Porter (1997). Reprinted by permission of HarperCollins Publishers Ltd © Roy Porter, 1997.

Chapter 2 epigraph:
Wildavsky (1997) © 1977 by the American Academy of Arts and Sciences. By permission of MIT Press Journals.

Chapter 4 epigraph:
Douglas and Wildavsky (1983). Reproduced by permission of The University of California Press.

Chapter 6 epigraph:
Zola (1978/1972: 501). Reproduced with permission.

Figures

Figure 2.1: Office for National Statistics (2006) *Social Trends*. London: HMSO. Crown copyright 2006. Online Edition.

List of Contributors

Stephen Bowler is currently researching a book on suffering and subjectivity. Stephen has also contributed several essays on health at www.spiked-online.com.

Tracey Brown is Director of Sense About Science, a charitable trust promoting good science and evidence for the public. The trust's work aims to raise the standards of science in all areas of public life and covers a wide range of contentious issues such as chemicals, radiation, vaccines and genetic modification. Tracey is a regular contributor to public and media debates on science, the public and progress.

Alan Buckingham is Senior Lecturer at Bath Spa University. Alan has research interests in social inequality – particularly class inequality – and the social effects of welfare policy. He is co-author, with Peter Saunders, of *The Survey Methods Workbook* (Polity, 2004).

Adam Burgess is Senior Lecturer in Sociology at the University of Kent where he lectures on the historical sociology of risk. His last book, *Cellular Phones, Public Fears and a Culture of Precaution* (Cambridge University Press, 2003) was widely praised internationally. He is currently researching British public inquiries, and belief in 'drink spiking'.

Mike Bury is Emeritus Professor of Sociology at the University of London. He was head of the Social Policy and Social Science Department at Royal Holloway from 1996 to 2001. Mike's main research interests have been in the sociology of chronic illness and in ageing. More recently Mike has been concerned with self-care in chronic illness, and wider aspects of health policy and medicine. Mike's most recent book is *Health and Illness* (Polity, 2005). He has served on a number of public bodies including the MRC and NICE. Mike was the co-editor of *Sociology of Health and Illness* from 1995 to 2001.

Elizabeth Frayn is a specialist trainee in psychiatry, working in the NHS in London. She writes for www.spiked-online.com on medical matters, and has a particular interest in the impact of health awareness campaigns.

Frank Furedi is Professor of Sociology at the University of Kent. His research is oriented towards the study of the impact of precautionary culture and risk aversion on western societies. In his books he has explored controversies over issues such as health, children, food and cultural life.

Ellie Lee is Senior Lecturer in the School of Social Policy, Sociology and Social Research University of Kent. Her research engages the sociology of health and of the family. She is the author of *Abortion, Motherhood and Mental Health* (Aldine Transaction, 2003), and the editor of *Abortion Law and Politics Today* (Macmillan, 1998) and *Real Bodies* (Palgrave, 2002).

Vanessa Pupavac is a lecturer at the University of Nottingham. Vanessa's recent research examines the influence of western therapy culture on international aid policy and the rise of international psychosocial programmes. Her research is underpinned by an interest in contemporary subjectivity and the crisis of meaning in international politics. Vanessa was awarded the Otto Klineberg Intercultural and International Relations Award 2003.

David Wainwright is Senior Lecturer at the University of Bath. His research interests focus on the sociology of work and health. Previous publications have explored the social construction of the work stress epidemic, and he is currently researching the negotiation of health-related resilience within workplace social networks.

1

The Changing Face of Medical Sociology

David Wainwright

- Modern medicine has brought dramatic improvements in life expectancy and the treatment of disease.
- Despite these achievements medicine is increasingly viewed with suspicion and ambivalence.
- Medical sociology not only provides an analysis of medical discourse; its promotion of social models of health and illness have influenced the development of policy and practice.
- Three social models of health and illness are introduced and critiqued, concluding with an account of critical realism.

Medicine is an enormous achievement, but what it will achieve practically for humanity, and what those who hold the power will allow it to do, remain open questions.
Roy Porter, *The Greatest Benefit to Mankind*, 1997

The new discourse of health

The last century brought dramatic improvements in virtually all major objective indicators of health status, at least in the developed world. Many infectious diseases have been controlled, infant mortality has fallen dramatically and life expectancy continues to increase. The so called scourges of modernity, coronary heart disease and cancer, are slowly retreating in the face of high technology medicine. Science has ameliorated many of the more troublesome problems and constraints of the human body; reproductive technologies have radically extended control over fertility; transplant surgery has enabled damaged organs to be replaced; joint replacements have made the elderly mobile again; even the outward appearance of the body can be surgically manipulated and enhanced.

Yet despite these achievements there is a widespread belief that 'bio-medicine' is a double-edged sword. Rather than celebrating the benefits of modern medicine, many fear its potency, preferring 'natural' or 'complementary' remedies.[1] Rather than focusing on how rapidly medical science can be progressed and implemented, public debate is often concerned with subordinating technological innovation to legal and ethical regulation.[2] Scandals have erupted over the retention of human organs for research, and anti-vivisectionists have succeeded in placing the interests of animals ahead of those of humans.[3] New developments from stem cell technology, to gene therapy, to therapeutic cloning are presented as potential threats to be reined in and governed by the *precautionary principle*, which insists that safety must be proven before implementation – a demand which is arguably impossible to meet.[4]

Ambivalence about bio-medical science has been matched by a diminution of trust in health care providers, policy makers and other 'vested interests'.[5] The authority of the medical profession has been undermined by high-profile cases of professional incompetence or criminality. Clinical expertise and professional self-regulation are constantly eroded by a pluralistic approach to medical knowledge and the imposition of a managerial structure of control. Corporate interests, such as private health care providers and particularly the pharmaceutical companies are viewed with unalloyed suspicion. Neither the free market nor social planning are seen as legitimate means of advancing healthcare policy.[6]

The retreat from medical science has been matched by the promotion of a putatively social model of health and illness, based on two key observations: first that health status is shaped by social factors, for example, morbidity and mortality are patterned by social class, gender and ethnic group, and second, that health has a subjective as well as an objective dimension, that is, it is about how we feel and choose to act as well as the presence of physical pathology. Both of these observations are valid, but their translation into health policy and medical practice has brought adverse consequences.

Most notably, the emergence of the social model has radically expanded the domain of therapeutic intervention. Expenditure on health care may still be dominated by hospital services, but the thrust of health policy is much more towards the regulation of behaviour and the management of subjectivity. The New Public Health movement has shifted the clinical gaze from treatment of the sick to regulation of the well. What we eat, drink and smoke, who we sleep with, how we relate to family members and friends, and the demands of working life, have all become subjects of professional advice in the pursuit of that elusive endpoint: 'wellbeing'.

The regulation of healthy bodies has been matched by a rapid expansion of psychotherapeutic intervention. Most of the Victorian asylums have been closed and their inmates decarcerated, but the reintegration of the mentally ill has been accompanied by a blurring of the boundary between sanity and madness. New psychiatric and psychological categories have emerged, such as Attention Deficit Hyperactivity Disorder, Seasonal Affective Disorder, Post-traumatic Stress Disorder, and a host of new addictions, to pathologise what were previously thought of as aspects of everyday emotional life. The severely mentally ill may have to wait to access scarce psychiatric resources, but a burgeoning army of arguably underqualified and loosely regulated psychotherapists is available to minister to the anxious and the glum.[7]

Taken together the New Public Health and the rise of psychotherapy have led to a significant transformation of the relationship between the individual and the state. Aspects of everyday life which were previously sacrosanct have been opened up to therapeutic scrutiny and regulation. This colonisation of the lifeworld has given momentum to a new sense of personhood which emphasises vulnerability and dependence. Health scares which emphasise the physical or emotional threat posed by mundane aspects of everyday life, such as, sunbathing, using a mobile phone, work stress, vaccination, and so on are commonly reported in the media. Paradoxically, as health has improved, stoicism and resilience have declined. Physical and mental health are increasingly viewed as fragile states which need to be defended against a growing list of social and environmental threats.

The above trends and changes constitute a fundamental shift in our experiences of health and illness and constitute the emergence of a *new discourse of health*. The history of medical sociology parallels this transformation.[8] From the high water mark of clinical science in the post-war period, to the psycho-social model that informs much health policy today, medical sociologists have not been passive observers, simply documenting changes as they unfold, but have played a signifi-cant role in interpreting, and in some instances precipitating, change. Broader social, cultural and political forces have driven these changes, but medical sociol-ogy has often provided the crucible in which these changes are made sense of; for-mulating the language and analytical framework through which policy makers, professional elites and pressure groups have articulated them. Thus, many of the themes to be found in contemporary public debates about health have their origins in earlier sociological discourse; the social model of health now shared by many medical practitioners and policy makers has its origins in sociological accounts of the social causation of illness, and the critique of medical power to be found in many official reports damning clinical autonomy and calling for greater regulation of the medical profession can be traced back to the medicalisation thesis of the 1970s.[9,10,11,12]

The aim of this book is to explore these transformations by examining a series of key issues in the contemporary experience of health and illness from a sociological perspective. Our approach is not to see medical sociology as detached from its sub-ject matter, but to pick up on an earlier debate within the sub-discipline,[13,14,15] which recognises that medical sociology has played an active role in shaping that which it also reflects upon. A sociology of time would not begin by taking the back off a clock, but by observing the movements of the hands around the clock face and studying the social consequences of time-keeping. Likewise we begin our account of medical sociology not by 'taking the back off' to reveal its conceptual and methodological components, but by observing the changing face of medical soci-ology and its consequences for how society collectively makes sense of the experi-ences of health and illness.

The emergence of medical sociology

Writing the intellectual history of medical sociology presents several problems. The sub-discipline has drawn on perspectives and theories from mainstream sociology, including functionalism, symbolic interactionism, Marxism, feminism and post-modernism. Different paradigms have had more or less prominence at different points in time, for instance, Parsonian functionalism in the 1950s, interactionism in the 1960s, Marxism and feminism in the 1970s and post-modernism in the 1980s. However, although this crude chronology grasps something of the changes that have occurred in medical sociology, it needs to be treated with circumspection.

First, the rise and fall of the different paradigms does not reflect a linear process of scientific progress from error and ignorance to truth and knowledge, for instance, the apparent decline in the study of the political economy of health from the late 1970s and the growing interest in the epistemology of medical knowledge from the early 1980s, cannot be explained exclusively in terms of the inadequacies of the former or the veracity of the latter. Second, mapping paradigms onto specific periods of time implies a degree of homogeneity and consensus which is hard to find in reality. Not all medical sociologists writing in the 1950s were doctrinaire Parsonian functionalists; likewise the concepts and theories of feminism have influenced medical sociology across its history, not just in the 1970s. The influence of different perspectives varies not just across time, but also between countries, sociology departments and individual writers. Third, the researchers who have contributed to medical sociology are increasingly difficult to pigeon-hole in terms of the perspective that informs their work. Not only are they often drawn from disciplines outside sociology, but few define themselves exclusively as Marxists, feminists, interactionists or post-modernists. The influence of different intellectual traditions can still be observed, but they are often invoked and synthesised pragmatically according to the research question that is being addressed. This 'mix-and-match' approach is particularly apparent in empirical research, for example, proponents of 'mixed methods' often combine qualitative and quantitative methods of data collection, despite the difficulty of reconciling the epistemological assumptions of naturalistic and positivist methodologies.[16]

Finally, while medical sociology is a product of intellectual currents and methodologies drawn from mainstream sociology and applied empirically to the study of health and illness, their significance is only apparent behind the walls of the academy, in seminar rooms and lecture theatres, publications and conference proceedings. The face that medical sociology presents to the world and, more importantly, the influence that it has had on the way in which society makes sense of and comes to understand experiences of health and illness, is not mediated through the categories and constructions of different strands of social theory, but through engagement with a much broader discourse of health, specifically through the articulation of social models of health and illness.

Social models of health and illness

The bio-medical model of disease with its emphasis on physical pathology and biological reductionism has been criticised for neglecting the social influences on health and illness. While bio-medicine has advanced over the last century, a range of other disciplines including sociology, psychology, epidemiology and economics has explored these social influences on health, providing not just a critique of the limits of bio-medicine, but a different way of understanding and addressing health and illness. This *social model of health* is often presented as a single unified theory; however, the range of assumptions and perspectives included under this broad umbrella is so diverse that it is more accurate to refer to several social models. No taxonomy is likely to capture all of these differences, here we have aggregated them into three broad groupings which can be identified in the literature and which have had a significant impact on the broader discourse of health: the social determinants of health; unhealthy lifestyles; and the social construction of health and illness. It should be noted that there is inconsistency and disagreement within these groupings as well as between them.

The social determinants of health

This perspective has been adopted by epidemiologists and others working in the field of social medicine. Of the social models this is closest to the bio-medical model in that it is traditionally concerned with physical pathology, but seeks to extend notions of aetiology or disease causation, beyond the identification of a pathogenic agent, such as a virus, to include social and economic factors, such as poverty, homelessness and air pollution. This approach has a long history, charting the influences of urbanisation and industrialisation on the nation's health from the beginning of the industrial revolution.[17] Central to the approach is the claim that material deprivation plays a fundamental role in the causation of disease, as the poor are denied many of the goods and services required for health and are more likely to be exposed to environmental hazards, such as damp housing or occupational injuries.

The social determinants of health model is supported by a substantial body of empirical evidence which reveals a strong social gradient for most diseases, with the poorer classes experiencing higher rates of disease than their more affluent peers.[18] From this perspective social development, particularly reducing poverty, poor housing and environmental pollution, play a more important role in improving the nation's health than that played by curative medicine.[19] This claim has not gone uncontested.[20]

If evidence is required for the claim that an adequate supply of food and clean water, shelter from the elements, clean air and protection from hazardous substances and machinery in the workplace, make a significant contribution to health, then the contemporary experience of many people living in the third world will provide it. But what about societies in the developed world which have succeeded in providing these basic requirements for health; has rising affluence and the welfare state succeeded in overcoming the social determinants of disease? Evidence suggests that above a certain level of social development an *epidemiological transition* occurs in which the traditional diseases of poverty, particularly infectious diseases and malnutrition, are replaced by the diseases of affluence, such as cancers and heart disease.[21] Despite these changes, social variations in health status persist, so where does this leave the social determinants of health model?

The epidemiological transition has prompted a conceptual shift in the social determinants of health literature. While some continue to pursue the materialist approach of linking health inequalities to the direct effects of deprivation or exposure to hazards, this perspective has been largely supplanted by a second strand which argues that the psychological consequences of social inequality now play a more important role than material deprivation in the causation of disease. The Whitehall studies[22,23] explored the health status of different grades of British civil servants over time and found that the junior grades experienced significantly greater ill health, especially heart disease, than their more senior colleagues. Although the grades varied in seniority, none suffered the material deprivation experienced by the poor, the implication being that the variations in health must be caused by the different psychological characteristics of the work done by different grades of staff. The second Whitehall study explored this possibility and found that junior staff reported higher job demands, lower job control and less social support at work than their senior colleagues.[24] Controversially, it was argued that exposure to these job characteristics caused psychological stress, which in turn triggered physiological changes which led to higher rates of disease. New disciplines, such as psychoneuroimmunology and ecocardiology have emerged to study the link between psychological stressors and disease, and more significantly, using international comparative data, Wilkinson has argued that beyond a certain level of economic development rich countries with wide economic inequalities have poorer average health than more equitable societies that have less wealth, because of the adverse health effects of psychological distress caused by social inequality.[25]

The claim that psychological distress can cause physiological changes in the body which in turn cause diseases such as heart disease, reduced immune function, or even some cancers, marks a fundamental shift in the social determinants of health model, which as we shall see in Chapter 4, has influenced the broader discourse of health. Introducing psycho-social stressors into the pathway between social conditions and physical pathology has revitalised the social determinants model and broadened its explanatory range in developed societies. However, its claims have not gone uncontested. The fundamental problem is that the social determinants model overlooks the subjective nature of psychological distress. While polluted water supplies or insufficient nutrition have an objective effect on the body irrespective of what the individual makes of their circumstances, this is not the case with psycho-social stressors which must be subjectively recognised and appraised as a threat in order to have an effect on the body.[26]

The problem becomes apparent in the social determinants of health literature on work-related stress. There are two dominant theoretical models in this approach to work stress or job strain: Karasek and Theorell's Demands-Control-Support model,[27] and Siegrist's Effort-Reward Imbalance Model.[28] Both models assume that work stress and the illness behaviour produced by it are an unmediated response to objective conditions in the workplace. For Karasek and Theorell the key factors are high job demands, low job control, and lack of support from other employees, and for Siegrist a disparity between the amount of effort invested in work and the rewards that are received is the trigger for the stress response. Missing from both models is any attempt to explain how people's attitudes and beliefs about what constitutes a heavy workload, or what is a reasonable reward for work, shape their response to their working conditions, or, how these attitudes and beliefs are shaped by personal experiences and changing cultural norms. This deficiency in the social determinants model leaves its proponents struggling to explain variations in the response to objectively similar working conditions between individuals and over time. Why do some people thrive in jobs which others find unbearably stressful, and why was work stress unheard of before the 1960s despite the physically and psychologically harsh working conditions that prevailed in the nineteenth and early twentieth centuries?

Unhealthy lifestyles perspective

Where the social determinants model underplays personal volition in the genesis of illness behaviour the unhealthy lifestyles perspective focuses on individual choices. Social variations in morbidity and mortality are recognised, but they are explained in terms of 'lifestyle choices', for example, the higher prevalence of smoking, alcohol consumption, dietary fat, and lack of exercise among the manual working class is seen as the primary cause of their higher rates of cancers and heart disease.[29]

The claim that lifestyle choices could have an impact on health and illness received much of its impetus from the groundbreaking research into the association between tobacco smoking and lung cancer by Austin Bradford Hill and his colleagues in the early 1950s.[30] The link between smoking and cancer was only confirmed after years of meticulous and highly rigorous research, yet the profound consequences of this research for the prevention of disease provoked the scientific equivalent of a goldrush as epidemiologists raced to find other Pathogenic Lifestyle Factors, often with far less caution and rigour than that employed in the search for a link between smoking and cancer.

A key moment came in 1981 with the publication of Richard Doll's *The Causes of Cancer*.[31] Doll had worked with Bradford Hill in the 1950s and, with his colleague Peto, added much to our understanding of the link between tobacco and cancer. As an internationally renowned cancer epidemiologist, Doll's claim that (excluding those caused by smoking) 70 per cent of cancers are caused by diet, carried considerable weight with policy makers, particularly as costly high-technology cancer treatments were making little headway against the disease. The notion that the pain, suffering and medical costs caused by cancer could be largely avoided simply by changing what we eat was compelling, but not without its critics.

Doll's argument in *The Causes of Cancer* is supported by a wealth of references and statistical evidence, but as Le Fanu[32] has pointed out, the basic methodology is a simple one. Essentially, his argument is based on comparison of specific cancer rates obtained from the Connecticut Cancer Registry, with the lowest recorded rates for those cancers elsewhere in the world, for example, Doll found 60 cases of pancreatic cancer per million head of population in Connecticut, compared with a mere 21 per million in India; a difference which Doll ascribes to the western diet which is heavy in high fat meat and dairy produce. Le Fanu points out that while diet may explain these variations, the evidence supporting this hypothesis is not nearly as compelling as that for the link between tobacco and lung cancer; there are conceptual difficulties, including the strong evidence that cancers are caused by ageing, and examples which contradict the dietary hypothesis:

> The Mormons and Seventh-Day Adventists are identical in virtually every way: they lead sober lives, don't smoke or drink and go to church on Sundays. The only difference is that the Mormons eat meat and the Seventh-Day Adventists on the whole are vegetarians. If the 'high fat diet' explanation for cancer was valid, the meat eating Mormons must *by definition* have a higher incidence of these cancers than the Seventh-Day Adventists. But they do not.[33]

Others have also pointed to the lack of scientific rigour in much of the epidemiological research on the relationship between lifestyle factors and disease, for instance, Skrabanek and McCormick[34] have argued that statistical associations between putative risk factors and health outcomes are frequently presented as cause-and-effect relationships even though these apparent associations could be caused by the effects of other factors which have not been controlled (confounding variables), or could even be produced by chance (Type 1 error). This and other criticisms made by Skrabanek and others are explored in greater depth in Chapter 2.

Despite a well-developed critique of the 'junk science' behind many of the claims made for the role of environmental and 'lifestyle factors' in the causation of disease, the epidemiological 'goldrush' continued to gain momentum, generating an ever increasing tide of 'health scares' about the potential threat to health and wellbeing posed by agents or substances encountered in everyday life, including: coffee drinking, hair dye, the use of phthalates in plastics, pesticide residues in fruit and vegetables, sunbathing, the MMR vaccine, formula baby food, mobile phones, oral contraceptive pills – the list continues to grow.[35] Such 'discoveries' make good news copy and are frequently reported in the media in highly sensationalised terms with scant regard paid to the scientific rigour of the research.

The unhealthy lifestyles perspective has also been criticised for *victim blaming,* because it implies that unhealthy lifestyle choices stem from irresponsibility or moral fecklessness and overlooks the extent to which choices are constrained by structural and cultural factors.[36] Not surprisingly, many in the social determinants of health camp have set out to debunk the unhealthy lifestyles perspective, by demonstrating the ways in which the choices of people living in poverty are constrained, for instance it has been argued that social security benefits are insufficient to support healthy eating.[37]

Another strand of the victim-blaming critique looks at cultural and psychological factors, for example suggesting that tobacco smoking and alcohol consumption are deeply embedded in working-class culture and that their use may be determined by peer-group pressure and the behavioural norms of the sub-culture.[38] Gender has also been presented as a determinant of lifestyle choices. The life expectancy of men is shorter than that of women, and it has been argued that men's higher mortality results from a culture of masculinity that values risky behaviour, including tobacco smoking and heavy drinking, and which discourages the uptake of health services and other health maintenance strategies.[39]

At the heart of this debate is an old tension between notions of free will and determinism. The unhealthy lifestyles perspective may (in early iterations) have overlooked socio-cultural influences, but it did at least credit the individual with a high degree of free will or agency, rather than viewing him as a pawn whose choices are pre-destined. The criticism that the unhealthy lifestyles approach is victim blaming is often founded on a far less optimistic assessment of human subjectivity. People's capacity to appraise the health risks of activities like smoking, weigh the likely costs and benefits, and *freely* choose how to live their lives, is often down-played in favour of a diminished sense of subjectivity in which individuals can never resist the influence of social determinants like peer-group pressure or stress. The assumption is that the individual cannot transcend his milieu and consciously choose a course of action which contradicts the script dictated by his social position.

The criticism that the unhealthy lifestyles perspective was victim blaming, emphasised the extent to which the approach initially overlooked structural and cultural influences on behaviour in favour of moral exhortation and stigma; however, the influence of this criticism has not been to shift attention away from the individual and towards tackling the social determinants of lifestyle choices, rather it has resulted in an approach which remains essentially individualistic but which emphasises the individual's diminished capacity to resist the external influences on behaviour. Where earlier strands of the unhealthy lifestyles approach assigned a significant role to personal choice and the individual's ability to assimilate evidence about the risks posed by unhealthy lifestyle choices, more recent approaches to the promotion of healthy lifestyles assume a diminished role for subjectivity, for example, the reluctance of some social groups to heed the evidence relating to the health risks of tobacco smoking, is increasingly explained in terms of the potency of the addiction and the individual's inability to resist social and cultural incentives to continue smoking.[40] As we shall see later, this has led to the development of a therapeutic approach to the promotion of healthy lifestyles which goes beyond the provision of health warnings to offer interventions which aim to bolster the individual's capacity to make the 'right' choice, for instance through the provision of nicotine patches to reduce the potency of physical addiction, or psychotherapeutic interventions to boost self-esteem or self-advocacy.

The unhealthy lifestyles perspective has also been applied to work-related stress. When work stress first began to emerge as an issue it was often applied to senior white-collar workers who, it was argued, were suffering from 'Executive Stress'. The assumption was that in vigorously pursuing career advancement by working long hours at the office and taking on a heavy workload and onerous responsibilities, such individuals were making themselves vulnerable to stress, burn-out and health problems such as ulcers and heart attacks. Popular culture in the 1970s contained several examples of former executives who had turned their backs on the 'rat race' in order to lead the 'good life'.

The implication is that choosing to work hard can be just as unhealthy a lifestyle choice as smoking or eating a high-fat diet. This theme is still apparent in debates about work/life balance which suggest that individuals need to adopt a healthy distribution of time and effort between the home and the workplace. This argument is often directed towards women who pursue a career but also want to have children or, in the language of popular culture, 'women who want it all'. It is often implied that such women are not only risking their own health and wellbeing, but also that of their children who are placed in nursery schools and childcare.

As with other examples from the unhealthy lifestyles perspective the claim that work stress is a consequence of personal choice is open to the accusation of victim blaming. Not everyone has the luxury of choosing how to divide their time between home and work, nor the freedom to determine their own workload. Again, the response of the unhealthy lifestyles perspective to such criticism has been to adopt a therapeutic approach to the stressed individual, for example through the provision of stress avoidance or relaxation techniques. Again, this stems from a diminished view of subjectivity; the belief that people lack the capacity to manage their own mental life without the support of professional intervention.

The unhealthy lifestyles approach represents an advance on the social determinants of health perspective because it recognises the role of subjectivity and individual choice in mediating the relationship between structural and cultural factors and illness behaviour. However, the way in which this process of mediation is conceptualised is simplistic and implies that unhealthy lifestyle choices either stem from lack of information about the risks associated with a particular activity or behaviour, or from a personal cognitive deficiency, which stops the individual from choosing a healthy lifestyle even when they recognise it as such. While the unhealthy lifestyles approach recognises that how we behave in the world is shaped by how we understand it and the choices we make that stem from this understanding, what it fails to grasp is the extent to which this understanding is not purely an individual affair but a product of social interaction and negotiation. This becomes apparent when we consider the third and final social model of health and illness.

The social construction of health and illness

Social constructionism is a means of conceptualising the way in which knowledge or *discourse* is produced and the effects that knowledge has on behaviour. The approach is based on the assumption that there is a gap between objective reality, how the world 'really is', and the ways in which that reality is represented in human consciousness. We are able to observe the real world through our senses, but the ways in which we label, understand and explain what we see are not simply a mirror image of reality but also the products of human interpretation, imagination and creativity.

Soldiers returning from war, for instance, may exhibit symptoms and behaviours which today might be labelled as 'Post-traumatic Stress Disorder' and, having received this psychiatric diagnosis, they might be provided with a range of thera-peutic services, excused from combat and perhaps given financial compensation. However, this way of labelling, understanding and responding to the emotional and behavioural problems of soldiers is not a unique or unmediated representation of objective reality, but a historically and culturally specific way of understanding and making sense of the phenomenon. In their account of military psychiatry in the twentieth century, Jones and Wessely[41] explore the different ways in which the same symptoms have been labelled and understood. During the Boer War soldiers whose emotional state rendered them unable to fight were diagnosed with 'Disordered Action of the Heart', a generation later in the First World War the same symptoms were labelled as 'Shell Shock'. During the Second World War, air crew who had lost the will to fight were diagnosed as suffering from 'Lack of Moral Fibre', not surprisingly many were reluctant to have their exhaustion and fatigue stigmatised in this way, although the phrase is perhaps preferable to the earlier 'Lack of Intestinal Fortitude'.

The shifting lexicon of military psychiatry represents much more than the appli-cation of new names to old problems. It is not just the label that changes, but the understanding and explanation of the symptoms, for example the labels discussed earlier variously locate the origins of mental distress in the heart, the gut or the psy-che. These different ways of understanding the phenomenon have implications for the self-identity of the individual so labelled and for the ways in which others respond to them. A modern soldier suffering from Post-traumatic Stress Disorder will feel differently about himself and be treated differently to a World War II air-man suffering from a Lack of Moral Fibre, yet both might be exhibiting the same symptoms and behaviour. Indeed, during the First World War many soldiers were executed because their mental distress was defined as cowardice.

The ways in which we make sense of phenomena, the words we use to label them, and the theories we develop to understand them, have fundamental conse-quences for the self-identity of the individual who experiences the phenomenon and also for the ways in which others respond. This approach was taken up in the 1960s by labelling theorists who explored the way in which 'normality' and 'deviance' were defined and enforced through the imposition of socially constructed labels. The key insight of labelling theory is that deviance is not seen as inherent in the behaviour of an individual, but dependent upon the imposition of a label by powerful others; as Howard Becker famously put it, 'deviant behaviour is behaviour that people so label'.[42] The value of this insight for medical sociology is immedi-ately apparent; it raises the possibility that the diagnostic categories and labels applied by the medical profession to their patients may be largely independent of physical pathology. Robin Scott in *The Making of Blind Men* explored the way in which visually impaired, but partially sighted, people were encouraged to relin-quish their efforts to use their remaining vision and take on the role and self-identity of complete blindness, through the process of diagnosis and labelling. He notes that 'the overwhelming majority of people who are classified as blind according to this definition [i.e. the Snellen measure] can in fact see'.[43]

Labelling theory raises the political question of which social groups have the power to impose a label and make it stick. In a classic social experiment Rosenhan[44] sent a group of volunteers to seek entry to 12 mental institutions in the United States. All of the volunteers reported a single symptom consistent with a diagnosis of schizophrenia: claiming to have heard voices in their head saying 'thud' or 'empty'. All of the volunteers were diagnosed as schizophrenic and admitted to hospital. Despite the fact that none of the volunteers were mentally ill and did not exhibit further symptoms, they were kept in hospital for up to 52 days. While many of their fellow patients detected their sanity, the psychiatric staff did not change their initial diagnosis and interpreted the volunteers' behaviour, for example the writing of field notes, as further evidence of mental pathology.

Rosenhan's study reveals the way in which expert knowledge, in this case psychiatry, is implicated in the labelling process, by providing an interpretation and a set of expectations which can be imposed on the individual, often against their best interests. For social constructionists, this insight applies beyond psychiatry, to a much broader discourse of medical knowledge, for example, in the early 1970s Ann Oakley[45] challenged the way in which childbirth was increasingly constructed as a medical procedure, dominated by high technology wielded by doctors, and in which the expectant mother played a largely subordinate if not passive role. Interestingly, Oakley's work gave impetus to the natural childbirth movement, whose promotion of home births, minimal pain relief, and breast feeding, is arguably just as disempowering as the medicalised model it seeks to challenge.

Social constructionists share a common belief in the gap between objective reality and the phenomenal forms or discourses through which reality is represented in human consciousness. Where they differ is in the extent to which they believe that this gap can be bridged by the scientific method. Among sociologists who apply social constructionism to the study of health and illness there is a divide between those who retain a *realist* orientation, which starts from the assumption that there is an objective reality which can be known by humanity even if this knowledge is vulnerable to distortion by social and cultural influences, and those who embrace *relativism*, in which science-based knowledge cannot be viewed as any truer than that derived from other belief systems, such as, Catholicism or homeopathy.

In the late twentieth century, epistemological relativism had a profound influence on British medical sociology, from those who were keen to elevate the lay perspective on health and illness:

> medical theories and lay theories are, from a sociological point of view, of equal interest and status. Magic, religion, politics, science, sociology, can all be seen as folk systems for understanding the world. They can all be taken equally seriously.[46]

to those intent on diminishing the status of bio-medical science:

> A body analysed for humours contains humours; a body analysed for organs and tissues is constituted by organs and tissues; a body analysed for psychosocial functioning is a psychosocial object.[47]

The notion that no belief system or discourse could claim to offer a truer account of reality than any other has practical implications, according to those who advocate *medical pluralism*. If bio-medical science has no epistemological primacy then why should its practitioners have a privileged position in the diagnosis and treatment of illness; why should the oncologist be preferred to the acupuncturist; why should the general practitioner's diagnosis be accepted more readily than the patient's account?

From this perspective, the production of medical knowledge or discourse is simply a means of justifying the exercise of power and the truth or falsity of that knowledge becomes an irrelevant issue. The claim that scientific knowledge is essentially concerned with the exercise of power rather than the pursuit of truth is central to the work of Michel Foucault:

> the problem does not consist in drawing the line between that in a discourse which falls under the category of scientificity or truth, and that which comes under some other category, but in seeing historically how effects of truth are produced within discourses which in themselves are neither true nor false.[48]

For Foucault, discourse is much more than a body of knowledge, it also includes institutions, practices and technologies, thus the discourse of psychiatry not only includes a set of beliefs and ideas about the functioning of the mind, but also the therapeutic regimes and other apparatus used in the governance of the mentally ill. Foucault's project was a historical one, to reveal how different discursive formations emerged over time, and their implication in the exercise of power; an approach which he applied to criminality, madness, sexuality and, in *The Birth of the Clinic*,[49] to medicine. Central to Foucault's argument is the claim that the 'clinical gaze', as it emerged in the hospitals of nineteenth-century France, did not simply *reveal* an objective physiological reality which had previously lain undiscovered, but that it simply *created* a new way of making sense of the body based on the techniques of surveillance and observation, but also bound up in the exercise of power. Of course, many others before and after Foucault have explored how social knowledge is used to serve the interests of the powerful. Marx's account of ideology claims that in any historical period the dominant ideas will be those of the ruling class.[50] However, there are key differences between the approach adopted by Foucault and his followers and others who have adopted a critical perspective on social knowledge.

First, where others see ideology as a distortion of objective knowledge, which can be penetrated to reveal an authentic and essential truth, for Foucault there can be no escape from discourse. Replacing one set of beliefs with another does not represent progress in the journey towards an objective account of reality and, to the extent that emancipation can be achieved, it lies in rejecting the authority of truth claims rather than in revealing their falsehood, for example while the discourse of psychiatry may be implicated in the social control of deviance, liberation lies not in replacing existing psychiatry with a discourse which more adequately grasps the reality of madness but in questioning the distinction between madness and reason and psychiatry's right to police the putative boundary between the two.

A second difference lies in Foucault's emphasis on the micro-relations of power. Rather than seeing power residing in institutions, such as the state, or in a dominant class, race or gender, Foucault sees power as something which cannot be accumulated but only exercised in specific situations, such as the doctor–patient relationship. Moreover, power is not exercised as repression but as a productive force, for example in *The History of Sexuality*[51] Foucault overturns the traditional view that the Victorian period was characterised by sexual repression, by pointing to an explosion of discourse on sexuality, producing new subjects, such as the masturbating child and the hysterical woman. It is this process by which discourse is internalised by the individual as a means of making sense of his own subjectivity, that Foucault aims to reveal, particularly in his later writings. It is not just the case that discourse legitimates the coercive actions which others exercise over the individual, but the extent to which discourse provides *technologies of the self*,[52] ways of reflecting on and understanding our sense of selfhood. Thus, for Foucault there is no pre-social self existing outside of discourse. While we may subjectively experience a sense of scepticism about different knowledge claims and critique or challenge them, the apparatus we use for this critique, be it rationalism, Marxism or psychoanalysis is itself socially constructed – while we have the illusion of being an independent critical thinker, we have only used one form of discourse to overturn another.

Not surprisingly, Foucault's bleak conclusions and those of other strong constructionists, have been challenged by critics in the realist camp. In the field of medical sociology Bury's[53] critique of strong social constructionism has been highly influential and has provoked considerable debate within the sub-discipline.[54] Bury's critique contains three key components. First, that social constructionism does not give sufficient weight to the lived reality of the body as it is experienced in everyday life; pain suffering and death are only too *real* for those touched by them. Second, Bury argues that strong social constructionists underestimate the demonstrable effectiveness of bio-medical interventions in preventing and curing disease. While mistakes have occasionally been made, and some of the improvements in health status that have occurred over the last century may be attributable to social development rather than clinical interventions, there remains a compelling body of evidence to show that the eradication of many infectious diseases, the amelioration of physical trauma, and many other improvements in mortality and morbidity rates are directly attributable to the practice of modern medicine. In response constructionists have argued that this body of evidence relating to the effectiveness of bio-medicine is itself a social construction which is specific to the time and culture in which it was produced.

This leads to Bury's third criticism, that the relativism adopted by strong social constructionists is self-refuting: if one belief system cannot be judged more valid than any other, then why should the claims of social constructionists be accepted as truthful. Nicolson and McLaughlin have responded by suggesting that social constructionists do not deny an individual's right to judge the truth or falsity of knowledge, only the claim that one belief system is truer than another. This defence has its flaws, however. When social constructionists state that their analysis debunks science's claim to grasp objective reality more adequately than other belief systems, they are surely saying that social constructionism is a more valid belief system than science. Also, just how are individuals supposed to judge the truth or falsity of knowledge if the evidence presented to support or contradict it must always be dismissed?

The relativist strand of social constructionism reached its high point in the postmodernism of the closing years of the twentieth century. More recently, a new strand of social constructionism has emerged in medical sociology, influenced by the *critical realism* of Roy Bhaskar and his followers.[55] The ability of the scientific method to produce knowledge which grasps objective reality more accurately than other belief systems is accepted, but it is also recognised that other social and cultural factors are bound up in the transition from rigorous scientific enquiry to the production of a scientific discourse.

There is of course, room for scientific debate and contradictory interpretations of data within the parameters of scientific enquiry. Moreover, scientific evidence can be strong or weak depending on methodological rigour and the number of times that an experiment or observation has been replicated. Thus scientific knowledge is never fixed or irrefutable; there is always the possibility that new observations or better data will lead to the revision or rejection of a scientific theory. Social and cultural factors can also intervene to bias or invalidate scientific research. More broadly, the decision to apply the scientific method to one area of study rather than another is also shaped by social, economic, political and cultural factors. Most importantly, the decision of how to respond to scientific evidence is shaped by the same non-scientific factors, for example the link between tobacco smoking and lung cancer is well supported by scientific evidence, but if and how to respond to this finding, whether to ban smoking, produce information leaflets for smokers, develop nicotine patches, or develop better treatments for lung cancer, or not to respond at all, depends upon far more than scientific evidence of the likely outcome of such responses.

Critical realism, therefore, entails an engagement with the scientific content of a discourse, but also a sociological critique of the political, economic and cultural factors that determine the form taken by a particular discourse at a specific point in time. Burgess's analysis of the health scare surrounding the use of mobile phones,[56] for example, comprises a thorough evaluation of the scientific evidence concerning the health risks associated with mobile phones. Having established that the scientific evidence of a health risk is very weak, Burgess goes on to explore the sociological factors that have given rise to the ongoing discourse of risk management and precautionary measures. The value of the analysis stems not from an outright dismissal of scientific evidence, but from the attempt to disentangle that in a discourse which is rigorously scientific and that which is socially constructed.

As with Foucauldian social constructionism, critical realism is also concerned with the ways in which discourse creates subjects and gives rise to particular forms of subjectivity. Wainwright and Calnan's[57] analysis of the work-stress epidemic, for example, critically engages the scientific evidence relating to the effects of paid employment on mental health and provides a sociological critique of the social and cultural forces that have shaped the work-stress discourse, but it also examines the consequences of medicalising problems at work rather than constructing them as political or economic problems. While the discourse of work-stress is presented as an objective scientific account of the psychological consequences of conditions in the workplace, the analysis reveals that the emergence of the passive work-stress victim is contingent on broader social and cultural factors, which give rise to this form of subjectivity.

Critical realism, therefore, neither takes scientific discourse at face value, nor does it dismiss its claim to grasp reality more adequately than other belief systems. Rather than overturning the scientific project, critical realism aims to complement and extend scientific rigour by revealing the social and cultural aspects of scientific discourse. The goal of this approach is to aid the development of *critical consciousness*, which synthesises the insights of scientific enquiry, with an awareness of the different ways in which scientific knowledge can be interpreted and applied to the resolution of problems and the fulfilment of human potential. Scientific discourse can never be reduced to a core of objective knowledge which is absolute and incontestable; there can be no *purely* scientific solutions to human problems and advancement, but critical realism can bring into consciousness the conjuncture between science, social and cultural distortions, and political will.

Conclusion

This chapter began by identifying some of the paradoxes, tensions and uncertainties that characterise the contemporary experience of health and illness in western societies which, taken together, represent the emergence of a distinctly new discourse of health. Objectively, our health is improving, but subjectively we have a heightened sense of vulnerability, risk and anxiety. While rates of objectively measurable physical pathology are in decline subjective symptoms and associated forms of illness behaviour continue to rise. Many of the improvements in rates of objective health indicators stem from the application of modern scientific medicine, yet the trustworthiness of the professions, institutions and organisations responsible for developing and delivering effective health care is increasingly being challenged. Medical sociology exists to understand and explain these changes, but is itself embroiled in them.

Medical sociology is in a constant state of flux. There is not a linear process of development charcterised by a cumulative accretion of knowledge, but a continual cycle of contestation in which different standpoints are adopted, challenged and tested against the reality of lived experience and the problems of everyday life. In this chapter we have considered three of the main strands of the social model of health and illness. While each strand has contributed substantially to our understanding of health and illness there are fundamental problems with each. They explain part of the human experience of health and illness, but leave unanswered questions relating to free will and determinism, the mind–body problem, science and discourse, individualism and collectivism, realism and interpretivism. There are no easy answers to any of these questions, and it seems unlikely that a grand unified theory lies in wait around the next conceptual corner. Even so, there is some evidence of a growing recognition of the limitations of earlier approaches and a willingness to develop new ways of thinking about health and illness that transcend these limitations. Critical realism is one such attempt, but it is important to recognise that this is not a fully extemporised theory in which all of these tensions are resolved; it remains very much a work in progress.

Discussion topics

- Why has the relationship between medical sociology and medical science often been an antagonistic one? Is this antagonism inevitable?
- Are the three social models of health compatible, complementary or antagonistic?
- What are the differences between strong social constructionism and critical realism?

Further reading

Bury, M. (1986) Social constructionism and the development of medical sociology. *Sociology of Health and Illness,* 5(1): 1–24.

The definitive repost to the post-modernist turn in medical sociology and a forthright assertion of the need for sociological critique to be grounded in realism.

Gerhardt, U. (1989) *Ideas about Illness: An Intellectual and Political History of Medical Sociology*. London: Macmillan.

Charts the development of medical sociology from 1950 to the mid 1980s. Comprehensive and detailed.

Le Fanu, J. (1999) *The Rise and Fall of Modern Medicine*. London: Little Brown & Co.

An inspirational and highly readable account of the 'twelve definitive moments' that comprised the clinical science revolution, coupled with a critique of the social model and the new genetics.

Strong, P.M. (1979) Sociological imperialism and the profession of medicine. *Social Science and Medicine,* 13A: 199–215.

A classic account of the tension between medical sociology and its subject matter and the spark for an ongoing debate in the discipline.

References

1 Cant, S. and Sharma, U. (1998) *A New Medical Pluralism? Complementary Medicine, Doctors, Patients and the State*. London: Routledge.
2 Miller, P. and Wilsdon, J. (2006) *Better Humans? The Politics of Human Enhancement and Life Extension*. London: Demos.
3 Elston, M.E. (1994) The anti-vivisectionist movement and the science of medicine. In J. Gabe, D. Kelleher and G. Williams (eds), *Challenging Medicine*. London: Routledge.
4 Calnan, M., Wainwright, D., Glasner, P., Newbury-Ecob, R. and Ferlie, E. (2006). Medicines next goldmine: Implications of 'new' genetic health care technology for health services. *Medicine, Health Care and Philosophy*, 9: 33–41.
5 Allsop, J. (2006) Regaining trust in medicine: Professional and state strategies. *Current Sociology*, 54(4): 621–36.
6 Wainwright, D. (1998) Disenchantment, ambivalence, and the precautionary principle: the becalming of British health policy. *International Journal of Health Services*, 28: 407–26.
7 Wessely, S. (1996) The rise of counselling and the return of alienism. *BMJ*, 313: 158–60.
8 Gerhardt, U. (1989) *Ideas about Illness: An Intellectual and Political History of Medical Sociology*. London: Macmillan.
9 Freidson, E. (1970) *The Profession of Medicine*. New York: Dodd Mead.
10 Illich, I. (1975) *Medical Nemesis*. London: Calder & Boyars.
11 Illich, I. (1977) *The Limits to Medicine*. Harmondsworth: Penguin.
12 Kennedy, I. (1981) *The Unmasking of Medicine*. London: Allen & Unwin.
13 Strong, P.M. (1979) Sociological imperialism and the profession of medicine. *Social Science and Medicine*, 13A: 199–215.
14 Strong, P.M. (1984) Viewpoint: the academic encirclement of medicine. *Sociology of Health and Illness*, 6: 339–58.
15 Williams, S.J. (2001) Sociological imperialism and the profession of medicine revisited: where are we now? *Sociology of Health and Illness*, 23(2): 135–58.

16 Johnstone, P.J. (2004) Mixed methods, mixed methodology health services research in practice. *Qualitative Health Research*, 14(2): 259–71.

17 Davey Smith, G., Dorling, D. and Shaw, M. (eds) (2001) *Poverty, Inequality and Health in Britain 1800–2000: A Reader.* Bristol: Policy Press.

18 Marmot, M. and Wilkinson, R.G. (eds) (1999) *Social Determinants of Health.* Oxford: Oxford University Press.

19 McKeown, T. (1976) *The Role of Medicine: Dream, Mirage or Nemesis?* London: Nuffield Provincial Hospitals Trust.

20 Colgrove, J. (2002) The McKeown Thesis: A historical controversy and its enduring influence. *American Journal of Public Health*, 92(5): 725–9.

21 Wilkinson, R.G. (1994) The epidemiological transition: from material scarcity to social disadvantage? *Daedalus*, 123(4): 61–77.

22 Marmot, M.G., Shipley, M.J. and Rose, G. (1984) Inequalities in death: specific explanations of a general pattern. *Lancet,* May: 1003–6.

23 Marmot, M.G., Davey Smith, G., Stansfeld, S.A. et al. (1991) Health inequalities among British civil servants: the Whitehall II study. *Lancet,* 337: 1387–93.

24 Marmot, M.G., Bosma, H., Hemmingway, H., Brunner, E. and Stansfeld, S. (1997) Contribution of job control and other risk factors to social variations in coronary heart disease incidence. *Lancet,* 350: 235–9.

25 Wilkinson, R.G. (1996) *Unhealthy Societies: The Afflictions of Inequality.* London: Routledge.

26 Lazarus, R. and Folkman, S. (1984) *Stress, Appraisal and Coping.* New York: Springer.

27 Karasek, R. and Theorell, T. (1990) *Healthy Work: Stress, Productivity, and the Reconstruction of Working Life.* New York: Basic Books.

28 Siegrist, J. (1996) Adverse health effects of high effort/low reward conditions. *Journal of Occupational Psychology*, 1: 27–41.

29 Fuchs, V. (1974) *Who Shall Live? Health, Economics, and Social Choice.* New York: Basic Books.

30 Doll, R. and Bradford Hill, A. (1954) The mortality of doctors in relation to their smoking habit. *BMJ,* June: 1451–5.

31 Doll, R. and Peto, R. (1981) *The Causes of Cancer.* Oxford: Oxford University Press.

32 Le Fanu, J. (1999) *The Rise and Fall of Modern Medicine.* London: Little Brown & Co.

33 Ibid., p. 354.

34 Skrabanek, P. and McCormick, J. (1989) *Follies and Fallacies in Medicine.* London: Tarragon Press.

35 Fitzpatrick, M. (2001) *The Tyranny of Health.* London: Routledge.

36 Crawford, R. (1977) You are dangerous to your health: the ideology and politics of victim-blaming. *International Journal of Health Services*, 7(4): 663–80.

37 Blackburn, C. (1991) *Poverty and Health: Working with families.* Milton Keynes: Open University Press.

38 Lewis, O. (1967) *The Children of Sanchez.* New York: Random House.

39 Lee, C. and Owens, R.G. (2002) *The Psychology of Men's Health.* Buckingham: Open University Press.

40 Townsend, J. (1995) The burden of smoking. In M. Benzeval, K. Judge and M. Whitehead (eds), *Tackling Inequalities in Health.* London: King's Fund.

41 Jones, E. and Wessely, S. *Shell Shock to PTSD: Military Psychiatry from 1900 to the Gulf War*, Maudsley Monographs 47. Hove: Psychology Press.

42 Becker, H.S. (1963) *Outsiders: Studies in the Sociology of Deviance.* New York: Free Press.

43 Scott, R.A. (1969) *The Making of Blind Men*. New York: Russell Sage.
44 Rosenhan, D.L. (1973) On being sane in insane places. *Science*, 179: 250–8.
45 Oakley, A. (1976) Wisewomen and medicinemen: changes in the management of childbirth. In J. Mitchell and A. Oakley (eds), *The Rights and Wrongs of Women*. Harmondsworth: Penguin.
46 Calnan, M. (1987) *Health and Illness: The Lay Perspective*. London: Tavistock.
47 Armstrong, D. (1994) Bodies of knowledge/knowledge of bodies. In C. Jones and R. Porter (eds), *Reassessing Foucault: Power, Medicine and the Body*, London: Routledge, p. 25
48 Foucault, M. (1980) *Power/Knowledge: Selected Interviews and Other Writings 1972–1977*, edited by Colin Gordon. Brighton: Harvester, p. 118.
49 Foucault, M. (1963) *The Birth of the Clinic: An Archaeology of Medical Perception*. London: Tavistock.
50 Marx, K. and Engels, F. (1845/1932) *The German Ideology*. Available online: www.marxists.org
51 Foucault, M. (1979) *The History of Sexuality, vol. 1: An introduction*. London: Allen Lane.
52 Foucault, M. (1988) The political technology of individuals. In L.H. Martin, H. Gutman, and P.H. Hutton (eds), *Technologies of the Self: A Seminar with Michel Foucault*. London: Tavistock, p. 146.
53 Bury, M. (1986) Social constructionism and the development of medical sociology. *Sociology of Health and Illness*, 5(1): 1–24.
54 Nicolson, M. and McLaughlin, C. (1987) Social constructionism and medical sociology: a reply to M. Bury. *Sociology of Health and Illness*, 9(2): 107–26.
55 Collier, A. (1994), *Critical Realism: An Introduction to Roy Bhaskar's Philosophy*. London: Verso.
56 Burgess, A. (2004) *Cellular Phones, Public Fears, and a Culture of Precaution*. Cambridge: Cambridge University Press.
57 Wainwright, D. and Calnan, M. (2002) *Work Stress: The Making of a Modern Epidemic*. Buckingham: Open University Press.

2

Doing Better, Feeling Scared: Health Statistics and the Culture of Fear

Alan Buckingham

- Health statistics show improvements in objective measures of health and longevity yet, paradoxically, there is a growing sense of fear about illness and an increase in subjective health complaints.
- The methods and statistical techniques employed in mapping the relationships between social factors and health outcomes often serve to amplify perceptions of risk, thereby contributing to the promotion of *health scares*.
- These methods and techniques are critiqued and their contribution to health scares such as obesity, passive smoking and HIV/AIDS is explored.
- The amplification of health risks is discussed in the broader context of sociological theories of the *risk society* and the *culture of fear*.

If most people are healthier today than people like themselves have ever been, and if access to medical care now is more evenly distributed among rich and poor, why is there said to be a crisis in medical care that requires massive change? If the bulk of the population is satisfied with the care it is getting, why is there so much pressure in government for change? Why in brief, are we doing better but feeling worse?

Aaron Wildavsky, 1977

The citizens of western nations have never enjoyed such good health. The control of infectious diseases and other medical advances means that we can expect to live many more years than our great grandparents. But, there is a problem. While we may be living longer, we feel increasingly worried about our health and vulnerable to illness. This has been described as the 'paradox of health'.[1] The sense of fear generated by these worries can, in turn, be seen as a cause of the increase in subjective illness and medically unexplained symptoms (see Chapter 5).

Health scares about everything from mobile phone masts to flu pandemics fill the newspapers, giving rise to a heightened sense of physical and mental vulnerability. As worries about our health increase, the burden on the health service has also increased. A significant proportion of the General Practitioner's (GP) workload comprises patients with symptoms that cannot be medically explained. Anecdotal evidence suggests that the 'worried well' are filling GPs' waiting rooms and jumping queues in order to get the flu jab.[2,3]

This heightened sense of fear is often given succour by government, for example the AIDS campaign of the 1980s painted a picture of an impending epidemic of heterosexually transmitted AIDS unless 'safe-sex' protocols were adopted. More recently, the government has mounted a new campaign about the risk of contracting HIV among heterosexuals and the need to practise safe sex, even though the evidence suggests that most of the recent increase in HIV/AIDS cases can be explained by HIV-positive people coming to the UK (mainly from Africa) and being diagnosed once here.[4]

Since the 1980s the number of health scares seems to have risen exponentially, including those linking oral contraceptive pills with thrombosis, and the link between obesity and a range of health problems including diabetes. The public are frequently urged to change their behaviour, to be vigilant and take precautions. However, in many cases the risks are small and the campaigns merely serve to further heighten fears among the well.[5] Programmes of health promotion and preventive medicine are often based on poor-quality or contested evidence. Even well-established programmes, such as screening for breast cancer, can be questioned, with the latest evidence suggesting that it may not save lives and may lead many women to undergo unnecessary treatment.[6]

How did we get to this position, where the sense of fear around our wellbeing is so out of touch with the empirical reality? We begin by examining objective and subjective measures of health, before examining the ways in which the statistical methods employed in epidemiological research can give a grossly misleading picture of health risks.

Measuring health and illness

Objective measures: 'doing better'

Until the beginning of the twentieth century males and females born in the UK could expect to live just 45 and 49 years respectively. Thereafter, life expectancy increased rapidly reaching 77 years for men and 80 years for women by the end of the century.[7] Mortality rates, which had remained fairly stable for hundreds of years, fell markedly during the twentieth century (Figure 2.1).

A large proportion of the drop in the mortality rate can be attributed to the drop in infant mortality. In 1901 about a quarter of all deaths occurred in those under 12 months old. By the turn of the millennium, this had dropped to below 1 per cent.[8] Improved sanitation, nutrition and the advances of modern medicine have reduced the risk of early death, not least by controlling infectious diseases (Figure 2.2). This increase has been bolstered by improvements in the treatment of coronary heart disease and some cancers. For Le Fanu, these statistics mark one of the greatest of human achievements: 'we are citizens of a society in which, utterly uniquely for the first time in history, most people now live out their natural lifespan to die from diseases strongly determined by ageing'.[9]

Most objective measures of morbidity and mortality show that our health has improved rapidly over the last 100 or so years, however, there exists an extraordinary paradox in all of this for in recent years increasing evidence seems to suggest that we feel less well.

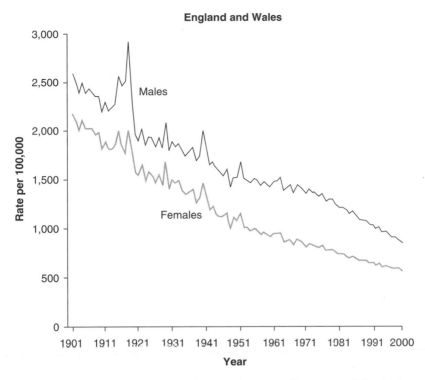

England and Wales

Figure 2.1   Age-standardised annual mortality rate, all causes of death, by sex, 1901–2000[10]

Source: Office for National Statistics (2006) *Social Trends*. London: HMSO. Crown copyright 2006. Online Edition.

Subjective measures: 'feeling worse'

In contrast to the sharp drop in organic illnesses and increase in life expectancy across western societies, subjective medical complaints have become increasingly common. A recent study of the Norwegian population found that within the previous month, 75 per cent had experienced musculoskeletal pain (including 47% reporting back pain), more than 50 per cent reported tiredness, 47 per cent gastrointestinal problems and 29 per cent an allergy.[11] When given a list of 25 possible somatic symptoms, men claimed an average of 2.8, and women an average of 3.9, symptoms in the last month.[12] In other research, 81 per cent of college students reported having at least one somatic symptom in a 3-day period.[13] Cases of people with a collection of somatic symptoms have also become commonplace, with nearly a third of women reporting 5 or more concurrent symptoms and more than 1 in 20 reporting 12 or more concurrent symptoms.[14]

Research estimates that in around a third, and possibly as many as four-fifths, of cases of reported somatic symptoms, no organic explanation can be found.[15,16] The prevalence of medically unexplained symptoms has serious consequences for medical resources. Between 25 and 50 per cent of all primary care consultations

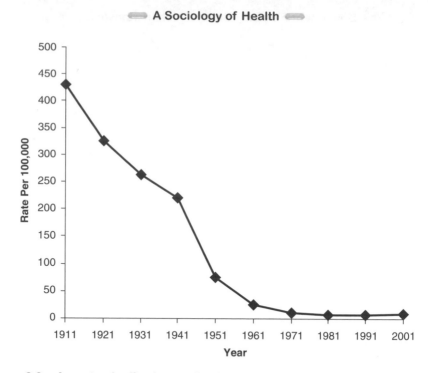

Figure 2.2   Age-standardised mortality rates caused by infectious diseases in England and Wales, 1911–2001[17]

Source: Adapted from Griffiths, C. and Brock, A. (2003) 'Twentieth Century Mortality Trends in England and Wales', *Health Statistics Quaterly*, 18: 5–17. Crown copyright 2003. Online edition.

involve patients presenting medically unexplainable symptoms, while the rate among specialist consultations is estimated at between 20 and 40 per cent.[18,19] In the Netherlands, functional somatic symptoms are now ranked second on the list of the ten most common physical symptoms presented to medical professionals in primary care.[20]

Self-report data show that 20 per cent of people in Europe report long-term illness or disability. In Britain the figure is over 25 per cent while in Finland it reaches nearly a third of the sample.[21] Other data show that the proportion reporting ill health has increased substantially over the last 20 or so years, even controlling for the increasing age of the British population.[22]

Paralleling these data has been the 'discovery' and then medical classification of a range of subjectively defined illnesses where no organic cause can be found, such as irritable bowel syndrome, fibromyalgia and post-viral fatigue syndrome. Typically, these syndromes are constituted by remarkably similar symptoms, most of which also have no organic explanation.[23] These complaints account for an estimated one-quarter to half of all new medical outpatient consultations.[24]

Finally, such feelings of unwellness have also fed into behaviour. Currently over 2.5 million people in the UK are economically inactive and in receipt of state incapacity benefits due to a health-related problem. Among the working population, the sickness absence rate is currently around 3 per cent while within the civil service it has reached 4.5 per cent, accounting for over 10 days lost each year per employee.[25,26] In other countries the picture is very similar. In Norway, for example, the total number of recorded sickness days has increased by 65 per cent between 1996 and 2003 and the number receiving disability pension has increased by 26 per cent during the same period. Taken together, it amounts to no less than 'an epidemic of common health problems (worry, sadness, back pain, etc.) among people in receipt of income benefits and those who consult their practitioners'.[27]

Health statistics and the amplification of risk

Many have argued that the media play an important role in generating an atmosphere of fear and vulnerability through the regular diet of health scares and over-reporting of minor health risks.[28,29,30] While the media may be apt to inflate and exaggerate risks there are some who argue that the science on which these reports are often based is also a culprit.

In the view of writers such as Skrabanek[31] and Brignell,[32] a great deal of this research is little more than junk science; the methods are frequently suspect and morality rather than science is often the dominant driving force in the research. The results usually go unchallenged and are important in providing justification for government action in regulating social behaviour. Before examining some of the methodological issues in the production of health statistics, we first examine the notion of *risk factors*.

The obsession with studying risk factors

In the past many of the threats and hazards we faced were perceived as 'natural', that is, they came from our inability to control the natural world. However, Beck[33] argues that we now live in a *risk society* where the chief threats we face are the product of human activity – they are created by us, for instance, through environmental pollution, and global terrorism. In the view of Giddens,[34] while we have created a world of man-made threats, in modern societies we also have the capability to measure them and do something about them.

The precautionary principle is one such way in which possible hazards are assessed and it is now the dominant principle by which risk is judged in areas such as the environment and health.[35] The principle is essentially conservative because its default position is that precautionary measures should be taken unless it can be shown that the particular activity poses no significant threat. It explains why seemingly innocuous things like hanging baskets and doormats are sometimes prohibited by over-zealous local authorities because they are said to pose a theoretical risk to health.[36] Sometimes referred to as the 'better safe than sorry' principle, it works in practice by placing the burden of proof on showing that there is no threat. Evidence of even a potential risk is enough to invoke safety measures. The rise of the precautionary principle has given a strong imperative to the search for health risk factors, which can be controlled in order to prevent the onset of disease.

The ability to seek out medical risks has improved substantially in recent years due to a number of scientific and technical advances including the increased availability

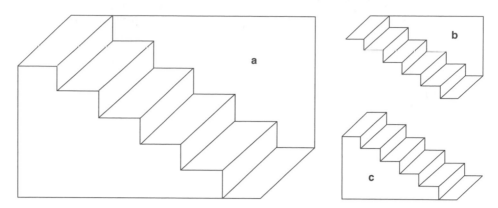

Figure 2.3   Data are always interpreted, but not just as we choose

of large datasets, advances in statistics used to describe and analyse data, and vastly increased computing capacity which allows data to be analysed quickly and cheaply. While this has allowed genuine and significant health risks to be identified, the techniques have also given rise to an 'epidemic' of weak or spurious relationships between social/lifestyle factors and illness. We now turn to the dubious methodological practices that have given rise to these spurious claims and to the health scares that have developed from them.

Misleading use of risk ratios

How researchers choose to present their data can have a powerful effect on our understanding of their findings. While we cannot make data say what we like, certain interpretations can be favoured through the way the data are presented. To understand this, take a careful look at Figure 2.3 and diagram A. At first you will probably see a staircase viewed from above. However, if you keep looking at the diagram you may find that your interpretation of the image switches. Now you will be seeing the staircase from below. Now take a look at diagram B and then C and you will see that the removal of a few lines can be crucial in influencing your interpretation of the image. In diagram B it now seems quite obvious that you are viewing the stairs from underneath while in diagram C it looks like you are viewing the stairs from above. The omission of a couple of lines in diagrams B and C has helped us make our mind up about how to interpret the diagram.

This example shows that facts are always interpreted by our brains and do not exist independently of how we look at the world. Observation, therefore, depends on our interpretation. This does not mean that we are free to interpret facts in any way we choose and that there is no objective knowledge. No matter how hard we look at the diagrams, we cannot see what is not there (you will not be able to see a tree or a boat, for example) and we would all have to agree on certain things present in the picture (for example, it consists of a series of straight lines). However, interpretations can vary and, depending on the way that facts are displayed, differing interpretations can be favoured.

What this means in terms of the presentation of scientific evidence is that, while researchers cannot make us believe what is not in the data, they can influence our interpretation by choosing different ways to display the data. Let us take the example of risk. The distinction is often made between scientifically established objective risk and perceived risk[37] as a way of separating the 'true' risk from our possibly inflated sense of risk. While useful, this distinction ignores the fact that the objective scientific risk can be reported in different ways and therefore perceived in different ways.

When describing risk, depending on the descriptive statistics used, two quite different pictures, one highly negative and one more positive, can be produced. The negative picture emerges if we choose a relative measure known as a *risk ratio*. This is the dominant way of describing social risk factors and works by comparing the risk of one outcome with the risk of another outcome across two different groups. Take for example the data on tobacco smoking and lung cancer. The typical comparison made is between heavy smokers and non-smokers in their chances of dying from lung cancer. Doll and Bradford Hill found that heavy smokers had a 24 times greater risk of dying from lung cancer than non smokers, that is, the risk ratio is 24 to 1.[38]

The risk of contracting lung cancer from tobacco smoking appears to be enormous and, indeed, subsequent research has yet to show any social or lifestyle behaviour which comes close to smoking in respect of the relative risk of death. However, the perception of risk is quite different if we consider the *absolute risk* rather than the *relative risk* expressed in a risk ratio. The fact that smokers are 24 times as likely as non-smokers to develop lung cancer might give the impression that most smokers will die from lung cancer, in fact, 16 per cent of male smokers and 9.4 per cent of female smokers contract lung cancer – while 90 per cent of lung cancers are caused by smoking, most smokers will not contract lung cancer. This still amounts to thousands of avoidable deaths per year, and there are of course many other smoking-related illnesses to consider; our point is simply that risk ratios can lead to an increased perception of risk.

This amplification of perceived risk is even more apparent when other examples are considered. Despite a regular diet of media stories about the effects of passive smoking and government bans on public smoking in many western countries, the relative risk (risk ratio) is tiny compared to that of a smoker dying from lung cancer. Instead of being 24 more times at risk from lung cancer than non-smokers (2400 per cent greater risk), passive smokers are about 1.24 times more at risk than non-smoke inhalers (24 per cent greater risk).[39]

A 24 per cent greater risk may sound large but, in absolute terms, the annual risk of dying from lung cancer for a person regularly exposed to secondary tobacco smoke is just 0.008 per cent. The absolute risk from passive smoking is so small, if it exists at all,[40] that it is difficult to measure accurately and is of no practical relevance. In addition, the findings are further undermined because a low-risk ratio like the one between passive smoking and lung cancer suggests a weak relationship, one that could easily be accounted for by error or some other third 'confounding' variable'.[41]

The one-sided and often inflated sense of hazard that risk ratios can portray has recently been recognised by an international committee set up to improve epidemiological research. It therefore recommends that absolute as well as relative differences should always be reported.[42] Despite this, absolute measures rarely make an appearance in research papers. It would seem that risk ratios, unsullied by absolute measures, are just too attractive to those who are signed up to the precautionary principle. The consequences for the non-specialist is that without the context of knowing the absolute risk, it is easy to become obsessed with the minute risks often portrayed in risk ratios and become obsessed with building one's life around avoiding any action that might increase the (relative) risk of ill health.

Risk by extrapolation

A further way of heightening risk awareness is by extrapolating data, for example, when the dire health effects of administering huge doses of a substance, (often in experiments on animals), are used as evidence that the substance is dangerous to humans, even though humans are only likely to consume tiny quantities of the substance. The logic that operates is that if a substance can be shown to be harmful, then regardless of dose – *ceteris paribus* – it must be a harmful substance. The problem with this is that, given a large enough dose, everything is harmful and given a small enough dose nothing is harmful.

A large number of environmental scares are based upon the fallacy of risk by extrapolation. It is well known that in high doses radiation can be harmful to health causing, among other things, leukaemia. Some years ago a cluster of cases of leukaemia near the nuclear reprocessing plant in Sellafield led to claims that leaking radiation from the plant had caused the cases. However, the exposure levels due to the plant were found to be far less than everyday recorded background levels to which we are all exposed and a minuscule proportion of the amount required to cause leukaemia.[43]

The same is true for a host of environmental factors alleged to be responsible for illness. For example, recent analysis of the radiation emissions from phone masts indicates that they are *hundreds* or *millions* of times below international guidelines.[44] Man-made pesticides in foods have been claimed to be carcinogenic but this is only in very high doses and the daily quantities we consume are tiny.

A second type of extrapolation involves drawing long lines of prediction based on trends of the last few years. Brignell[45] calls this the 'virtual body count' because trends extrapolated forwards produce larger and more scary numbers than can be found in the present data. Sometimes the historic data on which the trends are based only constitute a few years. The problem with this analysis is that it is akin to driving a car by only looking in the rear-view mirror; it is very difficult to predict the future based on scant evidence about the past.

One example of the misuse of trend data comes from a recent Department of Health-funded report examining future trends in obesity in England. This study made big headlines in the British press in 2006: 'England to Have 13m Obese by 2010' ran one headline and, inevitably, such is the imminent threat before long the text of the news story turns to the issue of government action and the banning of junk food advertisements.[46] The study itself attempts to predict levels of obesity in 2010 based on data recorded between 1993 and 2003 for adults and 1995 and 2003 for children. In the case of children the report predicts the prevalence seven years into the future based on just eight years of previous data. Knowing so little about past trends makes it likely that the forecasts will be inaccurate, especially when the past data are without a clear trend. For example, examining the year-by-year data for boys and girls on which the predictions are based, in only 2 of the 8 years was there a significant increase in obesity. These two years therefore account for virtually all of the overall upward trend in obesity between 1995 and 2003 and it is these two years that produce the upward trend in obesity that leads to the 2010 projections. Take away these two years and there is no upward trend in obesity.

Risk by definitional fiat

Inevitably we must impose our own categories on the world in order to be able to make sense of the chaotic and disorganised world around us. Science does this through classifications based upon a systematic taxonomic schema which groups things according to similarity in some respect. The division into groups or classes is usually based on some fundamental, categorical difference (for example, the existence of a backbone creates the classificatory division between vertebrates and invertebrates). Even in areas where the divisions are less clear-cut, scientists try to use rational, logical principles and argument to create categories. However, a significant amount of research into social risk factors is unconcerned with the technicalities of classification and the rigour it involves. Definitions are often arbitrary, lacking any clear rationale, and are liable to change.

The debate about obesity is a good example of the use of untheorised, arbitrary definitions. Obesity has been argued to be a risk factor in numerous diseases, from arthritis to sleep disorders.[47] The definition of obesity usually rests on the Body Mass Index (BMI), calculated by dividing weight by height squared. While some have questioned its ability to accurately measure excess fat, others have criticised the way in which arbitrary BMI thresholds are chosen to define people as 'underweight', 'desirable/normal', 'overweight' and 'obese'.[48]

Currently, the World Health Organisation (WHO) defines 'overweight' as those with a BMI of between 25 and 29. However, the rationale for the figure of 25 kg/m2 has never been specified. In addition, over time the threshold has changed, generally moving to a lower figure and thereby increasing the number of people classified as obese. For example, in 1998 the National Institute of Health lowered the US threshold for obesity from a BMI of 27 to 25. Overnight, without a single extra hamburger needing to have been eaten, the change increased the number classified as obese in the US by 30 million. Recently the WHO has suggested that the threshold for 'overweight' among Asians should be reduced from 25 to 23 and the obesity threshold from 30 to 25. If the new obesity threshold were to be accepted, magically all Asians currently defined as 'overweight' would become 'obese'. By definitional fiat these people are now firmly part of the 'at-risk group'.

The Department of Health study on obesity trends referred to earlier is also interesting, because of the role entirely arbitrary classifications play in producing the apparently scary findings of an obesity epidemic. When making the forecast of obesity levels in 2010, the study fails to inform the reader that a large proportion of the predicted increase in obesity can be attributed to, not more people getting fat but, people moving between the entirely arbitrary division of 'overweight' and 'obese'. In the case of obese women, while great play is made of the forecast 5 per cent rise between 2003 and 2010, the 3 per cent drop in the proportion 'overweight' is given scant attention.

The study also uses different and entirely incompatible measures of 'obese' for adults and children meaning that it is impossible to compare rates. The way in which childhood fatness is defined is particularly interesting because it is a statistical creation, based on selecting children in the sample who were in the top 5 per cent of the BMI distribution as recorded in 1990. Why 1990 was chosen as the base year and why the 'fattest' 5 per cent were chosen to be defined as 'obese' is never explained.

The truth is that categories are often morally conceived rather than scientifically established. This is evidenced by the fact that the labels for categories often reveal the moralising tendencies of the researchers. The Department of Health report, for example, sometimes refers to those with a BMI of between 20 and 24 as being of 'desirable weight'. In other literature this category is referred to as 'normal' or 'healthy'. The implication is that the remaining groups are undesirable, not normal or unhealthy.

If only we could do away with the risk of dying ...

A fundamental but often overlooked fact is that we all die of something, be it an accident, disease or illness. Life expectancy has a finite, biological limit and, in western societies, we may be close to reaching this limit. Over three quarters of all human deaths occur in those over the age of 75 and for these people death is simply due to old age.[49]

The process of ageing inevitably increases our vulnerability to pathologies. Ageing precipitates many of the common causes of death and, since we have not yet been able to stop people from ageing, we must accept that many of the diseases associated with old age, such as cancer and cardiovascular disease, are inevitable. As is often remarked, advancing age is one of the most potent of all carcinogens. However, 'in the minds of policy-makers and many biomedical scientists, no one suffers or dies from ageing'.[50] Rather, it is always classified as a disease that is preventable.

Since we have to die from something and since we have largely removed the threat of death from infectious disease, we are increasingly likely to die of illnesses associated with old age. However, the inevitable increase in these age-related diseases is treated as a mystery and an increasing threat.[51] Imagine for a moment that we had somehow cured death from all illnesses – even age-related ones – then there would necessarily be a very large increase in deaths from accidents. This is not because the world would be becoming any more dangerous but because of the logical fact that as one major cause of death recedes another cause must fill the vacuum. The paradoxical effect of medical advances in reducing the cause of one illness is that it necessarily increases the risk of dying from some other illnesses.

A lack of understanding of this fundamental fact means that people feel increasingly worried about illness as the media and experts report 'mysterious' and 'inexorable' increases in the prevalence of certain age-related illnesses. This is illustrated by an article that recently appeared in *The Ecologist,* which makes the claim that, 'Today chronic illness afflicts nearly half of all Americans and causes three out of four deaths in the US ... Things were not as bad in the 1930s'. In fact, it is suggested that we should look to primitive societies for the key to wellbeing: 'many observers ... have reported a virtual absence of degenerative disease, particularly cancer, in isolated, so-called "primitive" groups'.[52]

The author of the article makes a fundamental error in not recognising that few people will ever contract age-related diseases like cancer in underdeveloped societies because, as WHO data show, the average life expectancy in some of the African countries the author refers to amounts to less than 45 years and they are unlikely to live long enough to be at risk from such diseases.

Spurious risks

With an estimated $105.9 billion spent on health research a year,[53] the potential to find new risk factors is enormous. However, the surfeit of studies brings with it the increased chance of producing spurious results. It is a generally accepted rule among scientists that results are not reported as significant unless they are at least 95 per cent confident that their findings are not chance findings. This, of course, leaves us with up to a 5 per cent possibility that the results of the study might be a chance occurrence.

The 1 in 20 chance that any one study might find an erroneous relationship in the data (a false positive) is increased substantially when similar studies are repeatedly conducted testing the same hypothesis. With the large amount of money available for research and the ease with which data can be analysed, it is often the case that research into a particular hypothesised risk factor is conducted not once but 10, 20 or 100 times. The problem in all of this is, study a hypothesised relationship enough times and, by chance alone, eventually a relationship will be found in one study.

This is not necessarily a problem if a balanced approach is taken, where the results from each new study are placed in the context of the results of previous studies. The problem, however, comes from *publication bias*. This is the tendency of researchers, journal article referees and journal editors to see positive results as inherently more interesting and worthy of report than negative results. In short, positive results are more likely to be submitted for publication, accepted for publication and reported in the media.[54] The upshot is that the public disproportionately get to hear about the studies reporting the link between some social or environmental factor and a disease, and not the studies showing no relationship.[55]

Black box research: correlation does not equal causation

Risk factor health research only establishes associations, not causes. It does this by establishing that an aspect of personal behavior or some social factor is associated with a health-related condition. As Skrabanek makes clear: 'Risk factors have nothing to do with causes. They are risk *markers*, but they are neither sufficient nor necessary to explain the risk'.[56] So, for example, owning a driving licence is a risk marker for death in a car accident but, as with virtually all risk markers, the driving licence does not explain the causal mechanism behind road deaths. However, this is exactly the logic by which the social theory of health operates. Having established the risk marker, it frequently follows that there are calls for controls or bans on it. This is analogous to banning driving licences to stop car accidents. Not only would such action be draconian, it would fail to deal with the underlying cause of car accidents.

Multiple risk factors

The tendency to accept multiple risk factors as likely causes for an illness is often a product of the untheorised way in which correlations are accepted without any reference to whether a plausible biological mechanism exists. There is rarely a reasoned hypothesis about cause and effect; associations are found and it is then usually declared that social or lifestyle factors 'x, y and z' are determinants of illness 'a'. A relationship is only intelligible when we can establish a coherent and believable reason for the relationship. As Weber made clear over one hundred years ago, 'If adequacy in respect of meaning is lacking, then no matter how high the degree of uniformity and how precisely its probability can be numerically determined, it is still an incomprehensible statistical probability'.[57] In other words, it is simply no good blindly looking for associations if we do not have a reasoned, coherent and believable theory about why they are associated.[58]

A clear illustration of this issue can be found in research suggesting correlations between diet and coronary heart disease. A number of studies have shown that in countries with diets low in saturated fats the rate of Coronary Heart Disease (CHD) is much lower than in countries with diets high in saturated fats. It has also been found that those individuals with high levels of recorded cholesterol have an increased risk of CHD over those with low levels of cholesterol. The belief in the causal role of saturated fat in CHD still influences government policy today, with the reduction of saturated fat intake being a key aim of the NHS-funded Health Development Agency. However, the mechanism by which saturated fat could cause CHD is not understood and, some quite obvious evidence makes the alleged causal chain somewhat implausible. First, CHD rose very rapidly in countries like the USA during the 1920s, 1930s and 1940s at a time when there is no evidence of a correspondingly rapid change in diet. Second, the 1970s and 1980s have seen very rapid falls in CHD in all western societies even though diet changed little during this period.[59]

Confounding variables

A large but unknown number of health-related risk factors we seem to face are simply spurious. This means that the claimed causal relationship between the lifestyle factor and the illness can be explained by some prior third factor. Take a widely reported recent article that appeared in the *British Medical Journal* claiming that obesity is a risk factor in dementia.[60] Apparently, people in their 40s defined as 'overweight' are 74 per cent more likely to develop dementia compared to those defined as being of 'normal weight'. Not only is this relationship quite weak, there is also good reason to think that it is spurious. In a response to this report a group of researchers suggested a fundamental flaw in the study's conclusion:

> Obese people visit a medical doctor more frequently. Because dementia was not assessed for all participants of the cohort, but only for patients with a medical visit, obese patients had a higher chance to be diagnosed with dementia. This is a serious methodological flaw that should be communicated to your readers.[61]

Therefore, the rather weak relationship between obesity and dementia, far from being causal, as was suggested in many media reports, in all likelihood can be explained by a third factor – the frequency of visits to the doctor. If you do not visit a doctor it is difficult for you to be officially labelled as suffering from dementia. If you do visit the doctor – as obese people are more likely to do – there is clearly a greater chance of being defined as suffering from dementia. Of course, the possible flaw in the study was never reported in the media.

Strength of relationship

In considering whether an association is causal or not, the strength of the relationship provides good evidence about the likelihood of a causal relationship. In strong relationships it is unlikely that the relationship is spurious such that some third confounding variable, undetected biases or chance could explain the relationship between the two other variables. Strong relationships, like the one between smoking and lung cancer show a very large difference in risk between smokers and non-smokers (a risk ratio of 24 to1, it will be recalled). The strength of this relationship suggests that smoking is likely to be a cause of lung cancer.

Weak relationships, on the other hand, are much more open to the possibility of the relationship being spurious: 'The smaller the effect sizes in a scientific field, the less likely the research findings are to be true'.[62] It is for this reason that the usual minimum risk ratio accepted as evidence of a possible causal relationship is not less than 2 to 1.[63,64] There are times when this strict level can be relaxed, such as when there is supporting biological evidence, but relax it too far and the researcher runs the risk of accepting spurious results. Lifestyle risk factor researchers, however, can often be found reporting risk ratios of less than 1.5 and, as we have already noted, in the case of passive smoking, risk ratios of 1.25 have been accepted as valid evidence of a causal link between environmental tobacco smoke and lung cancer.

The strict principles that have traditionally guided scientific evaluation of data – the need to demonstrate consistent, strong and theoretically informed relationships in order to establish a causal relationship – have clearly been substantially softened in lifestyle health research. Reflecting this, the *British Medical Association* recently argued for the relaxation of long-held methodological principles used to establish causation.[65] This reformulation is based on the precautionary principle for it argues that just because there is only weak, inconsistent evidence that lacks a plausible theory it does not mean we can rule out the possibility of a causal relationship – better safe than sorry. This is tantamount to opening the door to poor science. It is also a recipe for scaremongering since it implies that weak and possibly flawed findings should be considered seriously just in case they have some credibility.

Rubbish in rubbish out: the limitations of self-reported illness

The above criticisms of health statistics and epidemiological methods refer mainly to the ways in which the relationships between objectively measurable risk factors, such as smoking, obesity, and toxic substances, and objective measures of morbidity and mortality, are conceptualised and presented. However, the scope for misconception and error increases substantially when risk factors and health effects are not measured objectively, but in terms of people's subjective accounts.

The problem is that there is often a poor correspondence between people's self-reports of illness and objective evidence of physical pathology. While it is frequently the case that exposure to social stressors is associated with self-reported illness, the link between self-reported illness and mortality is not strong.[66] In fact, some research shows an inverse relationship between self-reported illness and mortality. For example, the US states showing the most rapid drop in the mortality rate over the last five years are also the states that tended to show the most rapid rise in the proportion of respondents reporting poor health.[67]

Seen in this way, self-reported data on health status have to be treated with suspicion, because *illness claims* may reflect lack of self-esteem, worry and vulnerability rather than the presence of physical pathology. This is supported by research which shows that a range of psychosocial factors correlate well with self-assessed poor health but not at all with mortality.[68] More specifically, McLeod et al.[69]

found a significant correlation between stress and self-reported cardiovascular morbidity but stress and cardiovascular mortality were not correlated.

Worry is a powerful predictor of self-reported ill health. Worried and vulnerable people are much more likely to report symptoms. In one study the key predictor for symptom complaints after pesticide spraying in the area was worry and anxiety about modern technology and health.[70] Another study, examining students, found that worries about modernity and vulnerability to outside threats correlated with higher levels of health complaints and greater use of medical facilities.[71] The authors reason that those who are more concerned about environmental threats are also more likely to process somatic information as signs of illness. If self-reports of health status are not a reliable indicator of actual physical disease, then no amount of statistical finesse can overcome their limitations in exploring the relationship between social factors and disease – 'rubbish' data must inevitably yield 'rubbish' findings.

Health statistics and the culture of fear

Taking the critique of epidemiological methods as a starting point it is tempting to ascribe the amplification of health risks a primary role in the development of the *risk society* or the *culture of fear*. However, having criticised the tendency to attribute causality to relationships which are merely associations, we must take care not to fall into the same type of error. The amplification of health risks may coincide with the culture of fear, but there are many other sociological factors implicated in the current age of anxiety. According to Furedi,[72] fear has become firmly embedded within our culture as a result of broad historical and political changes. The break-up of traditional forms of social solidarity and cohesion, has reduced the sense of security that comes from strong affiliation to a group. The failure and demise of transformatory political ideologies and organisations has diminished the belief in our collective capacity to humanise nature and adapt it successfully to our needs. Similarly, the use of technology in war coupled with examples of environmental damage resulting from the misuse of technology, has created a backlash against science, and a desire to 'return to nature'.[73] These factors have given rise to a diminished sense of personhood, which emphasises powerlessness and passivity, rather than the humanist belief in man's unique capacity to transcend nature through the application of reason and agency. The prevailing culture of fear stems from this belief that the world is beyond our control; that we are individually and collectively incapable of mastering nature.

Health scares contribute to the culture of fear, but they are also a product of it. For Furedi,[74] in an age where fear, fatalism and human vulnerability have taken hold, it is not surprising that we worry about small and insidious threats to our health. The medicalisation of many previously normal aspects of everyday life (for example, pain, distress and sadness) acts to further widen the net of illness (see Chapter 6). Many of these medicalised symptoms have no organic basis and are largely diagnosed on the basis of unreliable self-reported symptoms. Illness is such a worry that it has become part of our identity and many people make sense of their experiences by reference to a medicalised web of meaning. This is supported by the evidence that the experience of illness is rapidly becoming normative rather than exceptional, with large numbers of people considering themselves to be suffering from one or more symptoms. The culture of fear and the amplification of health risks are mutually reinforcing. The widespread sense of vulnerability lies behind both the desire to seek out and quantify even the most tenuous of health risks, and the tendency to water down the scientific criteria by which the significance of this evidence is judged. Once in the public domain, these often dubious claims serve to reinforce the sense of vulnerability that precipitated them, and the circle begins again.

Vulnerability also gives rise to a strong moral impetus to regulate behaviour. The Jamie Oliver school dinners campaign illustrates this drive to regulate, ban and generally control on behalf of the 'vulnerable'. The crusade has led to a host of rules being introduced around school meals and a ban on school vending machines. Government guidelines now set highly prescriptive rules about what children may or may not eat. In so doing, it has conveniently enabled 'the dumping of every other food prejudice into the mix'.[75]

Although most parents and children appear to have accepted the new regime without a murmur, those who resist by bringing in 'non-permitted foodstuffs' have been met with a tough response. The next step has been to monitor compliance with the regime by weighing and measuring children and assessing whether they fit within the 'desirable' BMI category.[76] The long-term implications of this are to socialise a generation of children into believing that the food they eat is a potential threat which must be constantly guarded against and subject to statutory surveillance and regulation. It is through these experiences that the vulnerable and incapable individual, who takes seriously every media-hyped health scare, is reinforced.

Conclusion

This chapter has argued that the methods and statistical techniques used to map and report the putative relationships between lifestyle and environmental factors, such as dietary fat or passive smoking, and various measures of illness and disease, often amplify the perceived magnitude of the threat to health. These findings are often whipped up into 'health scares' through sensationalised reporting in the mass media and occasionally by the hasty and ill advised introduction of precautionary measures by government agencies (see Chapter 4 for a detailed account of this process). Such health scares have done much to undermine our collective sense of resilience by promoting a heightened sense of mental and physical vulnerability. The cumulative effect is to conceptualise the body as a fragile organism encircled by dangerous hazards lurking in even the most mundane substances and activities encountered in everyday life.

Discussion topics

- Why is it that when most objective measures of health status are improving, more people than ever report suffering from a long-term illness or disability?
- When reading newspaper reports about an alleged new health risk identified by research, what should you look for to assess the validity of the study and the significance of the threat?
- Why are the culture of fear and the amplification of health risks considered to be mutually reinforcing?

Further reading

Brignell, J. (2004) *The Epidemiologists: Have They Got Scares for You!* London: Brignell Associates.

A highly readable and enjoyable critique of epidemiology's role in the creation of health scares.

Office for National Statistics (ONS) (2006) *Social Trends*. London: Palgrave Macmillan.

A key resource for health statistics and much more. It should be bedside reading for all sociologists.

Skrabanek, P. (1991) Risk factor epidemiology: Science or non-science. In *Health, Lifestyle and Environment: Countering the Panic.* London: Social Affairs Unit.

Skrabanek was the sternest and most compelling critic of risk-factor epidemology and in this publication he summarises his assault on its claimed scientific status.

References

1 Barsky, A.J. (1988) The paradox of health. *New England Journal of Medicine*, 318: 414–8.
2 Fitzpatrick, M. (2001) *The Tyranny of Health.* London: Routledge, p. 10.
3 Wainwright, M. (2006) Flu jabs may be rationed or late as vaccine supplies are delayed. *Guardian*, 2 October.
4 Browne, A. (2006) *The Retreat of Reason.* Lancing, MA: CIVITAS.
5 Fitzpatrick, M. (2001) ibid.
6 Gotzsche, P. and Nielsen, M. (2006) Screening for breast cancer with mammography. *Cochrane Database of Systematic Reviews*, p. 4.
7 Office for National Statistics (ONS) (2006) *Social Trends.* London: Palgrave Macmillan.
8 Griffiths, C. and Brock, A. (2003) Twentieth century mortality trends in England and Wales. *Heath Statistics Quarterly*, p. 18.
9 Le Fanu, J. (1999) *The Rise and Fall of Modern Medicine.* London: Abacus, p. 314.
10 Office for National Statistics (ONS) (2006) ibid.
11 Ihlebaek, C., Brage, S. and Eriksen, H. (2007) Health complaints and sickness absence in Norway, 1999–2003. *Occupational Medicine*, 57(1): 43–9.
12 Haug, T.T., Mykletun, A. and Dahl Alv, A. (2004). The association between anxiety, depression, and somatic symptoms in a large population: the HUNT-II study. *Psychosomatic Medicine*, 66: 845–51.
13 Reidenberg, M.M. and Lowenthal, D.T. (1968) Adverse nondrug reactions. *New England and Journal of Medicine*, 279: 678–9.
14 Haug, T.T., Mykletun, A. and Dahl, Alv, A. (2004) ibid.
15 Kroenke, K., Spitzer, R.L., Williams, J.B., Linzer, M., Hahn, S.R. and deGruy, et al. (1994) Physical symptoms in primary care: predictors of psychiatric disorders and functional impairment. *Archives of Family Medicine,* 3(9): 774–9.

16 Kroenke, K. and Mangelsdorff, D. (1989) Common symptoms in ambulatory care: incidence, evaluation, therapy and outcome. *American Journal of Medicine,* 86: 262–6.
17 Adapted from Griffiths, C. and Brock, A. (2003) ibid.
18 Bass, C. and Sharpe, M. (2003) Medically unexplained symptoms in patients attending medical outpatient clinics. In D.A. Weatherall, J.G. Ledingham and D.A. Warrell (eds), *Oxford Textbook of Medicine.* Oxford: Oxford University Press.
19 Barsky, A.J. and Borus, J.F. (1995) Somatisation and medicalisation in the era of managed care. *Journal of the American Medical Association,* 274(24): 1931–4.
20 Van de Lisdonk, E.H., van den Bosch, W.J., Huygen, F.J.A. and Lagro-Janssen, A.L.M. (1999) *Psychische en Psychiatrische Stoornissen: Ziekten in de Huisartspraktijk.* [Psychological and psychiatric disorders: Morbidity in general practice] Nijmegen: Elsevier/Bunge.
21 Eurobarometer (2003) *Health Food Alcohol and Safety: Special Eurobarometer 186.* Wave 59.0. Brussels: European Commission.
22 Gravelle, H. and Sutton, H. (2006) *Income, Relative Income, and Self-reported Health in Britain 1979–2000.* York: Centre for Health Economics.
23 Barsky, A. and Borus, J. (1999) Functional somatic syndromes. *Annals of Internal Medicine,* 130 (11): 910–21.
24 Sharpe, M. (2002) Functional symptoms and syndromes: recent developments. *Trends in Health and Disability.* Dorking: UNUM Provident, 15–22.
25 Barham, C. and Leonard, J. (2002) Trends and sources of data on sickness absence. *Labour Market Trends,* 110(4): 177–85.
26 Feeny, A., North, F., Head, J., Canner, R. and Marmot, M. (1998) Socioeconomic and sex differentials in reason for sickness absence from the Whitehall II Study. *Journal of Occupational and Environmental Medicine,* 55: 91–8.
27 Aylward, M. (2006) Beliefs: clinical and vocational interventions tackling psychological and social determinants of illness and disability. In P. Halligan and M. Aylward (eds), *The Power of Belief: Psychosocial Influence on Illness, Disability and Medicine.* Oxford: Oxford University Press.
28 Frost, K., Frank, E. and Maibach, E. (1997) Relative risk in the news media: a quantification of misrepresentation. *American Journal of Public Health,* 87: 842–5.
29 Brown, J., Chapman, S. and Lupton, D. (1996) Infinitesimal risk as a public health crisis: news media coverage of a doctor-patient HIV contact tracing investigation. *Social Science and Medicine,* 43: 1685–95.
30 Winters, W., Devriese, S., Van Diest, I., Nemery, B., Veulemans, H., Eelen, P., Van de Woestijne, K. and Van den Bergh, O. (2003) Media warnings about environmental pollution facilitate the acquisition of symptoms in response to chemical substances. *Psychosomatic Medicine,* 65: 332–8.
31 Skrabanek, P. (1991) *Health, Lifestyle and Environment: Countering the Panic.* London: Social Affairs Unit.
32 Brignell, J. (2004) *The Epidemiologists: Have They Got Scares for You!* London: Brignell Associates.
33 Beck, U. (1992) *The Risk Society: Towards a New Modernity.* London: Sage.
34 Giddens, A. (1999) Risk and responsibility. *Modern Law Review,* 62(1): 1–10.
35 Guldberg, H. (2003) Challenging the precautionary principle. *Spiked,* 1 July.
36 Town bans hanging baskets. *BBC News.* Council targets 'danger' doormats. *BBC News.*
37 Slovic, P. (1987) Perception of risk. *Science,* 236: 280–5.

38 Doll, R. and Bradford Hill, A. (1954) Mortality of doctors in relation to their smoking habits. *BMJ*, 26 June: 1451–5.

39 Hackshaw, A.K., Law, M.R. and Wald, N.J. (1997) The accumulated evidence on lung cancer and environmental tobacco smoke. *BMJ*, 315: 980–8.

40 Enstrom, J. and Kabat, G. (2003) Environmental tobacco smoke and tobacco related mortality in a prospective study of Californians. 1960–98. *BMJ*, 326: 1057.

41 Davey-Smith, G. (2003) Effect of passive smoking on health. *BMJ*, 326: 1048–9.

42 Strengthening the Reporting of Observational studies in Epidemiology (2005) *Checklist of Essential Items Version 3*. Available at, http://www.strobe-statement.org.

43 Le Fanu, J. (1999) *The Rise and Fall of Modern Medicine*. London: Abacus, p. 361.

44 Burgess, A. (2002) Comparing national responses to perceived health risks from mobile phone masts. *Health Risk and Society*, 4(2): 175–88.

45 Brignell, J. (2004) ibid.

46 England to have 13m obese by 2010. *BBC News*.

47 Leveille, S.G., Wee, C.C. and Iezzoni, L.I. (2005) Trends in obesity and arthritis among baby boomers and their predecessors, 1971–2002. *American Journal of Public Health*, 95: 1607–13.

48 Gard. M. and Wright, J. (2005) *The Obesity Epidemic: Science, Morality and Ideology*. London: Routledge.

49 Weon, B.M. (2004) Analysis of trends in human longevity by new model. *Demographic Research*, 27 January: 10.

50 Hayflick, L. (2000) The future of ageing. *Nature*, 408: 267–9.

51 Brignell, J. (2004) ibid.

52 Fallon, A. (2003) Nasty, brutish and short. *The Ecologist*, 1 July.

53 Global Forum for Health Research (2004) *Monitoring Financial Flows for Health Research 2004*. Geneva: Global Forum for Health Research.

54 Koren, G. and Klein, N. (1991) Bias against negative studies in newspaper reports of medical research. *Journal of the American Medical Association*, 266: 1824–6.

55 Copas, J.B. and Shi, J.Q. (2000) Renalysis of epidemiological evidence on lung cancer and passive smoking. *BMJ*, 320: 417–18.

56 Skrabanek, P. (1991) ibid.

57 Weber, Max (1947) *Max Weber: The Theory of Social and Economic Organization*. New York: The Free Press, p. 99.

58 Feinstein, A. (1998) Scientific standards in epidemiological studies of the menaces of daily life. *Science*, 242: 1257–63.

59 Le Fanu, J. (1999) ibid., pp. 328, 337.

60 Whitmer, R.A., Gunderson, E.P., Barrett-Connor, E., Quesenberry, C.P., Jr. and Yaffe, K. (2005) Obesity in middle age and future risk of dementia: a 27-year longitudinal population based study. *BMJ*, 330: 1360.

61 Janneke, N., Belo, J., Feleus, A. and van der Wouden, J. (2005) Association between obesity and dementia may be spurious. Available at: http://bmj.bmjjournals.com.

62 Ioanndis, J. (2005) Why most published research findings are false. *PLoS Medicine*, 2(8): e124.

63 Taubes, G. (1995) Epidemiology faces its limits. *Science*, 269: 164–9.

64 Ioannidis, J. (2005) ibid.

65 British Medical Association (BMA) (2004) *Smoking and Reproductive Life: The Impact of Smoking on Sexual, Reproductive and Child Health*. London: BMA.

66 Johansson, S.R. (1991) The health transition: the cultural inflation of morbidity during the decline of mortality. *Health Transition Review,* 1: 39–65.

67 Johansson, S.R. (1991) ibid.

68 Mackenbach, J.P., Simon, J.G., Looman, C.W. and Joung, I.M. (2002) Self assessed health and mortality: could psycho-social factors explain the association? *International Journal of Epidemiology,* 31(6): 1162–8.

69 Macleod, J., Davey Smith, G., Heslop, P., Metcalfe, C., Carroll, D. and Hart, C. (2002) Psychological stress and cardiovascular disease: empirical demonstration of bias in a prospective observational study of Scottish men. *BMJ,* 324: 1247–51.

70 Petrie, K., Broadbent, E., Kley, N., Moss-Morris, R., Horne, R. and Rief, W. (2005) Worries about modernity predict symptom complaints after environmental pesticide spraying. *Psychosomatic Medicine,* 67: 778–82.

71 Lind, R., Arslan, G., Eriksen, H.R., Kahrs, G., Haug, T.T. and Florvaag, E. (2005) Modern health worries in medical students. *Journal of Psychosomatic Research,* 58: 453–7.

72 Furedi, F. (2002) *Culture of fear.* London: Continuum.

73 Taverne, D. (2006) *The March of Unreason: Science, Democracy and the New Fundamentalism.* Oxford: Oxford University Press.

74 Furedi, F. (2003) *Therapy Culture: Cultivating Vulnerability in an Uncertain Age.* London: Routledge.

75 Lyons, R. (2006) The school meals revolution: a dog's dinner. *Spiked,* 9 November.

76 Obesity tests for four year olds. *BBC News.*

3

The Object of Medicine

Stephen Bowler

- What is specific to western medicine is a Cartesian view of health, in which mind and body occupy different realms of meaning. By contrast, a non-Cartesian view of health is the defining feature of 'complementary and alternative medicine', in which mind and body inhabit the same domain of enquiry.
- In treating disease as physical pathology, western medicine objectifies the human body. In so doing it acknowledges and reflects a distinction between biological apparatus and moral authority, as vested in a person's subjective state, which is, by turns, the locus of personal responsibility.
- This division of labour does not stand alone, and is ultimately legitimated at the level of society as a whole, where the aspiration to transcend the limitations of nature determines the value placed on medicine as an institution. The rise of 'complementary and alternative' medicine suggests a weakening of this aspiration.

Charlie Allnut: A man takes a drop too much once in a while, it's only human nature.

Rose Sayer: Nature, Mr. Allnut, is what we are put in this world to rise above.

The African Queen, 1951

The crisis in medicine and the rise of complementary therapies

Following the Public Inquiry into events at Bristol Royal Infirmary in the late 1980s and early 1990s, when paediatric cardiac surgery ran a 'flawed' service resulting in inadequate levels of care, the President of the General Medical Council, Sir Donald Irvine, observed how the 'self-confidence of the medical profession, and public confidence in the system of medical regulation, have been shaken to the roots by highly publicised clinical failures'.[1] Through the furore surrounding Alder Hey hospital in Liverpool, where body parts from child cadavers were routinely stored without consent,[2] to the striking-off of one of Britain's most eminent paediatricians, Professor Sir Roy Meadow (in July 2005) for having given evidence considered to be 'erroneous and misleading' in a murder trial, and on to the highly charged stand-off over the safety of the MMR vaccine,[3] modern medicine can be seen to have experienced an unprecedented challenge to its legitimacy. Unsurprisingly, doctors are reported to feel 'overworked and undersupported',[4] 'beleaguered' and 'perplexed'.[5] A 'growing feeling that altruism in medicine, if not dying, is at least declining' has been noted.[6]

At the same time as modern scientific medicine – also known as biomedicine – is experiencing a drop in confidence, both within and without, a rise in the fortunes of 'complementary and alternative medicine' (CAM) is evident. CAM 'has achieved an exponential growth over the last two decades. There is strong evidence of its popularity amongst users and this trend is particularly pronounced in the area of cancer'.[7] An estimated 19 million people use CAM in the UK,[8] where a 'notable increase in the number of ... patients who self-medicate ... with mineral and vitamin supplements over the last five years'[9] reflects a widening sympathy with its values. CAM now sits firmly within the mainstream of health care provision.[10] BSc degree courses in Homeopathy are now available within UK universities.[11] There are five homeopathic hospitals, fully funded within the NHS.[12] The 'NHS Directory of Complementary and Alternative Practitioners' sanctions a list of therapies from Ayurveda, Bodywork and Crystal Therapy through to Radionics and Reiki.[13] In the USA the market for CAM is 'huge and growing' and enjoys a rising legitimacy at the highest levels.[14] Clearly, the standing of medicine *per se* has not declined, only its specifically scientific version.

One way of understanding why one kind of medicine is waning and the other is waxing is to ask what medicine is for. Is the job of medicine to fix one's body when it breaks down, rather like a car, in order then to send us back out onto the highway of life, where we navigate our own way to our own chosen destination? Or is medicine more about the choice of destination, the wisdom of going there, and the kind of journey we might expect to have? Is the body an instrument to be used to achieve a goal – a means to an end – or is it a site of existence in its own right, which we should nourish and cherish? Is it a vehicle, or a temple? Do we need a mechanic, or a priest?

Here we explore this question, of the inter-relationship between medicine as an institution and our own inner expectations and needs as they are met – or not – by that institution. To the extent that the practice and priorities of modern scientific medicine mesh with our own subjective understanding of health and illness might it suit our needs and retain our confidence. Likewise with CAM, as an alternative paradigm to which many now turn. How we experience and enact our innermost aims and desires – our sense of person-hood or subjectivity – is intimately related to the kind of care and assistance we seek when things go wrong.

In order to understand how this works we need to unravel some basic concepts, and introduce some new ones. We need to step back from the inherently fuzzy concepts of sickness and health and assess the categories by which we make sense of them. We need, in particular, a clearer idea as to the object of medical care. Is it just the body, when it goes wrong? Or is its remit 'the whole person'?

Humanism and truth

In an insightful consideration of *What Is Specific to Western Medicine?*,[15] eminent American psychiatrist and anthropologist Arthur Kleinman stresses the 'monotheism of the Western tradition' that 'legitimates the idea of a single, underlying, universalizable truth'. This is a truth that can be grasped by all, rather than an elect few. One does not need a priest, shaman or healer to reveal it.

The truth of which Kleinman speaks is the wholly human capacity to exercise reason, the scientific method to which it gives rise, and the physical, organic nature to which it relates. It is monotheistic – that is, constructed in terms of a singular God – because deeply indebted to the Judeo-Christian tradition. Originally religious, this is, however, a debt that has long been paid off in 'the shift from the explicit religiosity of the scientific revolutionaries of the sixteenth and seventeenth centuries to the equally emphatic secularism of the western intellect in the nineteenth and twentieth'.[16]

It is hard now to appreciate that truth was once a quality handed down from on high – as Galileo found to his cost when trying to convince the Papacy that the Earth was not, in fact, the centre of God's universe, and the Sun was. We take for granted our capacity to think for ourselves, to question everything and seek out the inner logic and outer proof of a given proposition. But this is a faculty with a most particular story behind it, one that is synonymous with the broad church that is the western tradition, and the liberal-democratic norms of person-hood with which it is associated.

At 'a certain point in history men became individuals',[17] embracing the idea that we are each of us unique, with our own opinions, values and emotions and that each of us has a right to determine our own destiny in our own way. This was a dramatic departure from the experience of anyone living in the medieval era. And just as we might value our own individuality, so do we see this in others, recognising an essential sameness across humanity that would also have been unknown in premodern times.

This is the 'single, underlying, universalizable truth' of which Kleinman speaks. Once very much a narrative of God and His wisdom, it became, through the past two or three centuries or so, a wholly secular, irreligious truth, vested in the common human capacity to reason for oneself, and the 'celebration of objectivity and hardheaded commitment to fact'[18] to which it gave rise. Enlightenment was a movement in history that gave birth to science as we know it, but it was, more importantly, the time when men began to understand themselves in a radically new way, as agents of free will. It was 'both an idea and an *ideal* … a vision, often quite spiritually charged, of … a new time in which the world would be guided by reason and free of superstition'.[19]

Symbolic potency

What is specific to western medicine, then, is a historically novel way of seeing the world, constructed in relation to a 'single, underlying, universalizable truth' to which we all have access. All the techniques and tools and institutional trappings we spontaneously associate with medical science are ultimately products of this radically new kind of person-hood. Biomedicine is both an objectively identifiable set of practices, but also a subjectively comprehended understanding of those practices.

This is a complex point, but one that constitutes our key theme. It hinges on the psychological and emotional internalisation of a most particular way of defining the self, and how this outlook relates to the practice of scientific medicine. It is well addressed by Jonathan Miller in *The Body in Question*, where he considers the many and various ways in which disease has been understood over time, and how this is reflected in methods and beliefs about healing.[20]

Beginning with the observation that it is man – and man alone – who when sick 'is endowed with the capacity to reclassify himself as something in need of help', Miller moves on to consider the means by which this might happen. Throughout recorded history there have been healers, of one kind or another. To be successful a healer has to establish a particular kind of relationship with his audience. He must:

> identify himself with some principle which is popularly accepted as an authentic basis of medical control ... When an African villager submits to the regime of a local magician, he is impressed by the colourful drama with which the remedies are surrounded – by the mystery and the ritual and the esoteric confidence of the practitioner – but what sways him most is the fact that this particular type of healer acts upon the same principles of symbolic potency which the patient applies to every other aspect of his life.

Put otherwise, we can say that there is a correspondence between subjective expectations and objective practices – what might also be termed the 'specific plausibility structures'[21] underpinning the moment in question. Each element affirms the other in its symbolic unity. For the exchange to even take place the practitioner must connect with the inner expectations of the sick patient in terms of a shared universe of meaning. The 'same principles of symbolic potency which the patient applies to every other aspect of his life' constitute the grounds on which the therapeutic encounter takes place.

Whether modern or not, the observation that medicine is embedded in a symbolic order is persuasive. And to the extent that this order reflects what Miller calls 'one of the most basic assumptions of western medicine; namely, that all serious disease has an identifiable physical cause'[22] does it confirm Kleinman's view of western medicine as the product of a specific and systematic way of understanding the natural world, and man's place in it. Physical causes, after all, are only identified as such because mankind chooses, at a certain point in history, to name them that way – largely in the language of science. Doing so did not just change man's understanding of identifiable physical things on the outside; it also fuelled his own sense of purpose on the inside, as a creature with a future that could be consciously fashioned after his own interests.

In and through the scientific revolution (from mid-sixteenth to late seventeenth century[23]) this dynamic inter-relationship, between the possibility and the proof of change, underwrote the death of the old order and birth of the new. With the genie of human progress out of the lamp, a new narrative of the perfectibility of man inspired both the search for order in nature – in the form of scientific truth – and the confirmation of man's exceptional place in nature that was, and remains, the logical correlate of that activity. In the main this is a dynamic relationship that continues down to the present.

Take the discovery of helicobacter. Before the 1980s the dominant understanding of peptic ulcer was in terms of 'stress', and treatment reflected this view. But with the identification of helicobacter as the physical cause of peptic ulcer, a whole 'façade of knowledge' fell apart, provoking what James Le Fanu terms 'another "paradigm shift" in changing scientific understanding, not only of the diseases with which it is directly associated, but of all diseases'.[24] Confirmation that peptic ulcer had a distinct physical cause had the consequence of stripping this most commonly debilitating of diseases of its moral and behavioural connotations. In identifying and manipulating a tiny part of nature, scientific medicine confirmed a most particular view of nature, as authorised by that most unnatural of categories – man. Through rigorous experimental calculation, helicobacter was identified, analysed, and then neutralised, with the sole intention of enabling the larger organism that is the human body to flourish on terms that are strictly human. And if this is a 'negative' intervention, then consider a 'positive' in the form of the contraceptive pill; no less biologically complex, but even more significant as a tipping point from one paradigm of person-hood to another, enabling a whole generation of women to perceive of their potential in altogether more ambitious terms.[25] While the ultimate horizon of that ambition is not reducible to the medical technology, the 'feed back' of real, demonstrable benefits for whole populations reminds us of the cumulative and transformatory dynamic inherent in the drive for more and better methods of managing the human organism on terms that are more conducive to free willing human agency.

Mind and body

A useful way to begin to understand such themes is a report from a House of Lords Select Committee on Science and Technology[26] into the use of complementary and alternative medicine (CAM) that is 'widespread and increasing across the developed world'. Usefully, the report maps the various branches of CAM before asking what it is they share in common.

In contrast to the narrower biomedical focus upon 'elimination of symptoms and disease processes', CAM therapies attend to 'attributes such as good energy, happiness and a sense of wellbeing' as a way of 'strengthening the whole organism rather than directly attacking the pathology (such as an infection or tumour)', says the report. 'CAM therapies use different vocabularies to understand these emphases, with treatment concepts such as detoxification and tonification, and with different cultural concepts of "energy" as recuperative forces in the body'.[27]

CAM therapies attend to the whole person and not just their diseased part – their subjective experience as much as their objectively identifiable pathology. This 'holistic' emphasis is the key to understanding the 'different vocabularies' and 'different cultural concepts' deployed within CAM. All of which is in marked contrast to the biomedical approach, where it is the objective body – as opposed to subjective personality – that is understood as the site of pathology, and therefore the locus of therapeutic intervention. To return again to Arthur Kleinman: 'In the biomedical definition, nature is physical ... independent of perspective or representation ... The psychological, social and moral are only so many superficial layers of epiphenomenal cover that disguise the bedrock of truth, the ultimately natural substance in pathology and therapy'.[28]

In the words of the Select Committee, most CAM therapies 'apply a non-Cartesian view of health, making less distinction between the body, mind and spirit as distinct sources of disease. The language used in CAM often tends to imply that all these dimensions of the human condition should be viewed in the same therapeutic frame'.[29] Mind and body, such as Cartesian dualism separates, are reunited in CAM, the popular appeal of which lies in precisely this direction, 'satisfying a demand not met by orthodoxy'[30] by attending to the non-physical – subjective – dimension of modern person-hood.

A Cartesian view of health

In focusing upon the whole person, and not just their body, CAM 'applies a non-Cartesian view of health'. Put otherwise, we can say that biomedicine applies a Cartesian view of health. But what exactly does this mean?

To begin to answer this we need to step back in time and briefly note the name of René Descartes (1596–1650), the founder of modern philosophy and source of Cartesianism as a school of thought.

A devout Catholic his whole life, Descartes nonetheless established some of the key tenets of progressive thought in and beyond the Enlightenment. Chief among these, for our purposes, is his distinction between body and mind – hence Cartesian dualism – in which the former is considered in mechanical terms, as in any other animal, but the latter understood as divinely ordained soul. There was no other explanation for the unique and privileged place of man in the world of nature than the God-given capacity of men to exercise reason, argued Descartes. Brutes do not 'have less reason than men ... they have none at all'. Only man has a 'rational soul ... entirely distinct from body', and only man can wield that faculty to good effect. He ends his famous *Discourse on the Method* (1637) with a declaration to spend the rest of his life endeavouring 'to arrive at rules for medicine more assured than those which have as yet been attained'.[31]

In cleaving a 'rational soul' from a machine-like body Descartes made the case for knowledge as we understand it today, as conscious, reasoned, critically articulated insight. In bodily, organic terms man was no different to other animals. Indeed, in many respects he was less well adapted to his life than were the animals to theirs. But in one exceptional and precious sense he was blessed with an ability to stand back from nature, including his own, and hold blind evolutionary forces at arms length – to objectify them – in order to understand and mediate their impact.

Instead of a life fully engaged in nature, Enlightenment man sought to disengage himself from nature, the better to channel his passions more constructively and exercise his uniquely fertile intellect.[32] Our 'raging motions, our carnal stings, our unbitted lusts' are mercifully tempered by 'reason': were they not 'our natures would conduct us to most preposterous conclusions' wrote Shakespeare.[33] For the English philosopher John Locke (1632–1704), echoing the Cartesian wisdom of his day, it was man's ability 'to suspend the prosecution of this or that desire' that was the source of his liberty: 'in this seems to consist ... free-will'.[34]

A Cartesian view of health, such as biomedicine applies, is a dualist view of health. It is dualist in the fundamental assumption that mind and body denote two entirely different realms. One is the seat of our spirit, or self, that is reckoned in moral and intellectual terms, while the other is the form of our organic, natural existence. A physician could no more fix a damaged soul than a priest cure a hernia. In a strictly Cartesian world we seek out one kind of healer for one kind of problem, and another for the other. Free will consists in our ability to do both, as necessary.

A Cartesian view of health, such as biomedicine applies, is also an objective view of health. It orders and addresses pathology in relation to categories of disease that are universal, quantifiable and manipulable. Patients will have their own experiences of sickness, but doctors diagnose in terms of those common features that Arthur Kleinman describes as 'the bedrock of truth, the ultimately natural substance in pathology and therapy: biology as an architectural structure and its chemical associates'.[35] It is mathematics, rather than morality, that informs the scientific component at the heart of Cartesian biomedicine. This is not to say that medicine is an amoral enterprise, far from it: only that it has, in the main, been most successful when it has been most rigorously scientific, and therefore objective.

And finally, a Cartesian view of health is also a historical view of health. Just as the 'age of progressive optimism begins with the age of Descartes' medicine'[36] so is *The End of an Age of Optimism* signalled by the 'serious criticism of scientific medicine'[37] that arose in the late twentieth century. Put otherwise, the Cartesian view of health is inseparable from the Enlightenment optimism by which it was authorized. Peter Gay's characterization of scientific medicine as 'philosophy at work'[38] captures the proximity of ideas to practice. As 'an incomparable engine of analysis: objective, critical, progressive',[39] science powered the Enlightenment and the medicine that was its 'most heartening index of general improvement'.[40] And just as science was a broadly cultural as much as a narrowly technical quality from the time of Descartes through to the second half of the twentieth century, then so is it also contingent upon a wider progressive dynamic. The very qualities that made medicine valuable were also the qualities that made everything else valuable in the popular imagination.

These are complex and difficult themes. They tend to be the preserve of philosophy. But they are the key to understanding the distinction drawn by the House of Lords Select Committee between those therapies that apply a 'non-Cartesian view of health', and those that embrace the mind–body dualism of Cartesianism. What makes this distinction such a pressing and significant issue, though, is less a matter of medical technique than it is a representation of a wider cultural shift. As we have seen, it is not the authority of medicine *per se* that is waning, only its specifically Cartesian qualities. And in this consists the answer to our original question, of what medicine is for.

Before elaborating upon this, though, we should note some features of the 'non-Cartesian view of health'.

A non-Cartesian view of health

A non-Cartesian view of health is a holistic view of health, bringing mind and body within the same frame of enquiry. Within this frame there is a fusing of categories that remain distinct in biomedicine. The psychological, social and moral qualities that are placed aside in biomedicine – not because they are inconsequential for the patient, but because medical science cannot reliably objectify them – are placed centre stage in the therapeutic procedures of non-Cartesian CAM.

In bringing emotions, passions, and feelings into the diagnostic domain, CAM expands the meaning of health. Issues pertaining to a person's overall life course, and not just their pathologised physiology, are conceptualised in terms of energy, spirit, drives and forces. The narrative of care extends to the soul, or self, every bit as much as it extends to the body. Where scientific medicine seeks out facts, CAM works with values.

Perhaps the most significant value for CAM, as for any non-Cartesian outlook, is a view of nature as a beneficent, energising, and ultimately spiritual force in the life of man. In this it is in tune with one of the most influential strands of western thought – Romanticism. This is a rich and complex current that has played a decisive role in shaping how we perceive modern life in general, and science in particular. While individualism as we know it owes much to the idea of an autonomous and free-willing rational soul, or self, separated from one's own and other bodies, it has also come to be indelibly associated with the naturalist imagery of Romanticism and its ideal of earthy authenticity. In the words of one important text in this area:

> It is in literature and poetry that we first begin to encounter a reaction against Enlightenment values that reveals a specific distrust of science, as well as a strong reluctance to believe that mankind can be reformed along 'scientific' lines ... the poets [Blake, Wordsworth, Goethe] are linked by a strong commonality of thought. Each distrusts the narrowly empirical and the strictly rational, each celebrates the vital importance of the intuitive, the irreproducible moment of insight and of direct access to truth in its unmediated essence. Each accuses science, especially in its schematic mathematicized form, of blindness, or worse, stubborn refusal to see. Each fears a world in which scientific thought has become the sovereign mode, and recoils from the spiritual degradation and servility that, in his opinion, must inevitably come to characterize such a world.[41]

As the sovereign mode of health care in our time, biomedicine is indeed unsympathetic to intuition or insight. A Cartesian view of health deals in precisely those factors that can be defined in the most objective – scientific – of terms. 'Modern science, least bothered with the definition of human nature, knowing only the activity of investigation, achieves its profoundest results through anonymity, recognizing only the brilliant functioning of intellect',[42] observes the central character in Saul Bellow's archetypal modern novel, *Herzog*. The 'gilded age'[43] of clinical medicine in the post-war period, in which the novel is set, attests to the power of a mathematically grounded model of research, as well as a lot of state funding. This kind of hard, cold, impersonal, materialism, is though, for Arthur Kleinman, indicative of 'a thoroughly disenchanted world-view' where there is 'no mystery ... no magic at the core; no living principle that can be energized or creatively balanced'.[44]

The idea that biomedicine is 'a thoroughly disenchanted world-view' is significant. Clearly, medical science has no interest in magic or mystery. If enchantment means to fall under a spell, then modern medicine dispels and disenchants, recognising only such methods as can be shown to work. 'The dissecting blade of scientific scepticism' cuts away the mystery and insists that 'theories are worthy of respect only to the extent that their assertions pass the twin tests of internal logical consistency and empirical verification'.[45]

Romance, religion, and alchemy are alien to biomedicine. Where CAM focuses in upon the 'emotions, mind, attitudes and spirit of a total human being', for whom 'real health' is said to depend 'on the ability to express and be who [they] really are',[46] biomedicine displays an 'indifference to the experiences and emotions that make up life'.[47] Just as the mainstream of scientific thought says that 'knowledge obtained through scientific investigation does not in itself have a moral dimension',[48] then so does the mainstream of non-scientific opinion tend to promote precisely this dimension. The Prince of Wales, for example, a leading advocate of CAM, talks of a 'sacred trust between mankind and our creator ... that has ... become smothered by almost impenetrable layers of scientific rationalism'. We need, says Prince Charles, 'to rediscover a reverence ... a sense of humility, wonder and awe about our place in the natural order'.[49] We need, in other words, re-enchanting.

It is worth noting a central confusion of CAM, which immerses itself in the mystery of the very nature it reveres. It is in this respect thoroughly anti-transcendental, and stands in marked contrast to the Enlightenment origins of biomedicine, for which nature is a force outside of man, above which he seeks to rise. Put otherwise, we might see CAM as an expression of a diminished sense of person-hood, wherein reason is weakly conceived and takes the form of wishful thinking: 'positive thinking' is not uncommonly advocated as an approach to disease, as if the disease were a product of 'negative thoughts'. The consequence of this is a moralising of sickness and an intensification of anxiety.[50]

The changing object of medical care

We have considered two broadly opposed schools of thought with regards to the object of medical care, in terms of Cartesian and non-Cartesian views of health. The merits of this approach may not be immediately obvious – and may indeed seem rather complex – because of their historical and philosophical origins. It is, nonetheless, the distinction utilised by the House of Lords Select Committee, and the one explored here, for the simple reason that it cuts to the heart of the matter.

We have noted a relationship between mind and body, and the tension between a dualist and a non-dualist view of health. In a dualist view mind and body are two separate and irreconcilable categories: mind is immaterial, immortal, inorganic, subjective and value-laden, while body is material, mortal, organic, objective and value-free. Mind lends itself to intellectual, moral and spiritual enquiry while body lends itself to practical, scientific and rational enquiry.

As we have seen, this is a polarisation with a most particular pre-history. These are not timeless categories, but historical and relative to the sea change in human self-knowledge that was the Enlightenment. Mind relates to body as private relates to public, or self to society, in ways that are dramatically different from all preceding periods in history. But without an underlying tension to polarise these qualities they begin to lack meaning and can seem false. The dualism of Descartes and others, who put man at the centre of things by pushing nature to the margins, loses its dynamic, transformatory, transcendental edge. This is, arguably, where we are today.

Quite how we got here is a topic beyond this chapter, as is a consideration of 'underlying tensions' as drivers of human self-discovery. These are complex questions, well covered elsewhere.[51] Suffice to say, there is now wide sympathy for the idea that we should live, somehow, closer to nature. To be 'masters and possessors of nature', as Descartes once argued, has given way to a sense of ourselves as stewards of nature; a force with which we should co-exist, if not in harmony, then at least 'sustainably'. The critical distance between distinctively human interests and the rest of nature has narrowed, both in the cultural and political realm, but, more significantly, for our purposes, in the personal realm of health. It is this shift that begins to answer the question raised earlier, of what medicine is for.

Anti-dualism

The notion that modern man has travelled too far from his natural origins and needs to reconnect with them now sits in the centre of the western *zeitgeist*. Environmentalism is the key expression of this outlook, colouring all mainstream opinion a shade of green. What might be called the 'greening' of the body, as that part of nature for which one might entertain the deepest of reverence, and seek to act in the most sustainable of ways, has become a common theme – 'a return to Nature, through herbal remedies, natural cures, spiritualism, jogging and ginseng',[52] as Roy Porter once put it.

At the same time, though, we can identify a trend that seems to go in the opposite direction, toward a deeper probing of human biology in ever more technical terms. Every week we hear of new discoveries that link a particular gene to a particular trait, or reveal a place in the brain that determines a certain mood,[53] or claim to show the neurological origins of beliefs that might previously have been reckoned in wholly moral terms.[54] 'Morality is as firmly grounded in neurobiology as anything else we do or are', argues the primatologist Frans de Waal,[55] whose writing expresses an increasingly confident outlook on the part of evolutionary biology.[56]

What both these outlooks have in common is naturalism and a shared antipathy to Cartesian dualism as it has been discussed here. Authority resides in the raw data of natural forces in these perspectives, rather than the will of men. For sure, there is a world of difference between those seeking more mystery in nature and those wishing to decode it mathematically. But a rejection of the dualist distinction between an objectified physical body and a subjective agent of free will is one that is common to both. And at the heart of this rejection is a suspicion that free will is a dangerous illusion, used to justify an acquisitive and instrumental approach to nature on the one hand, or a raft of irrational and dogmatic prejudices on the other.

What has been squeezed out of the picture is freedom, as active self-knowledge. The 'idea of the individual human as a rational subject has taken a battering' observes Kenan Malik, 'because the idea of freedom has become degraded'.[57] While one might imagine freedom in abstract or formal terms, as human rights or parliamentary democracy, we refer here to that dimension of self that exists in a relationship of creative tension with the organic, physical self, and through this a relationship of creative tension with a wider natural order.[58] The unique capacity of man to reflect back upon himself and make his own history both reflects this creative tension and transforms it along the way. In objectifying and engaging with an external realm of nature, Enlightenment man forged a more rigorously critical and robust understanding of his own nature such as gave rise to modern scientific medicine.

But now we see a dimming of Enlightenment optimism and a near collapse in the idea of man as the measure of all things. Instead, man is now commonly understood as one part of a wider 'Gaia' – the 'complex entity involving the Earth's biosphere, atmosphere, oceans, and soil ... which seeks an optimal physical and chemical environment for life on this planet'[59] – wherein humanity is invariably considered a malign force. In which context the 'non-Cartesian view of health' – or anything else – begins to make sense, as unambitious existence, conscious more of the risks of change than the benefits of progress.

Being and having

The relationship between internal, existential aspirations and external, political possibilities is as broad as it is deep, and clearly beyond us here. We have acknowledged this vast philosophical terrain as the backdrop to the deceptively terse category of a 'non-Cartesian view of health' mentioned by the House of Lords Select Committee.

We have also painted biomedicine in fairly fundamentalist terms, neglecting to mention the various ways in which it does accommodate and address the subjective and qualitative dimension of patient care, from psychiatry to psycho-social medicine to the somatising disorders that are said to account for as 'many as one in five new consultations in primary care'.[60] Indeed, the story of modern medicine in the twentieth century is often told from this perspective, taking the many and various points of contact between biomedical authority and subjective experience as markers of medicine's ability to shape the innermost register of human health and shape the healing process. A fascinating literature on the placebo effect, for example, attests to the power and authority of medical science to harness the hopes and fears of patients to positive therapeutic ends.[61] Likewise, a rich strand of humanist writing on the subtleties and moral depth of the doctor–patient relationship attests to an understanding within medicine of its unique and privileged role in society.[62]

More prominent are texts that see the subjective and qualitative dimension of patient care in negative terms, either as a site of domination and control or neglect and indifference. If the former tends to be the preserve of medical sociology, the latter tends to be articulated in more mainstream circles. What both express is a deep unease with biomedical authority.

No less significant, though, are the various efforts from within biomedicine to refashion itself in the image of CAM, or, at least, to divest itself of the burden of the past and work toward a more 'patient-centred' model of care. It is important to understand that this does not simply mean more 'tea and sympathy' for the patient, but a clear downgrading of the authority traditionally accruing to a doctor by dint of his association with a more objective and rigorous domain of knowledge – science – than that available to the suffering patient. The inherent inequality of the doctor–patient relationship – in its traditional form[63] – is flattened and refashioned as a 'partnership ... based on mutual respect'.[64] In this it is entirely in tune with wider social trends, where the authority of expertise is commonly tempered by calls for 'the "public voice" to be brought into the formative stages of decision-making'[65] to facilitate the 'opening up [of] conceptual borders' that is thought 'key to achieving mutual understanding'.[66]

What we see, then, is less a polarisation of opinion, between Cartesian and non-Cartesian views of health, than a narrowing of the gap between them. This is what makes the Select Committee's distinction so useful, as ideal types that are themselves contingent upon the deeper, historically rooted paradigm of person-hood associated with the name of René Descartes. This is the demise of the Cartesian paradigm, not just in medicine, but more broadly too. To the extent that scientific medicine was popularly understood as the crowning achievement of modern rational thought then so did it confirm a dualist view of the body, and how it might be fixed in relatively mechanical terms. A strong streak of subjectivity in the life of an individual – or a whole society – reflected and enabled a strong streak of objectivity on the part of medical science. But where the creative tensions that push both sides apart are absent, the desire for more holistic practice arises.

Holism is an opaque concept with a chequered history:[67] 'essentially relational; it constitutes a rhetorical claim made in opposition to other approaches that are characterized as excessively narrow or reductionist in focus'.[68] This is the charge against the biomedical approach, and one often made in the form of the argument that 'health is more than the absence of disease'. The question is, though, 'how much more?'[69] At what point does health lose all meaning and become, instead, a register of everything as it impacts, or not, upon an individual? At what point does the individual become a product of all those forces, as opposed to a self-determining agent in his own right?

For such reasons have clinicians tended to stick with physical pathology, presuming in the main that a person's subjectivity is the moral property of the individual. Classically – from the earliest days of Enlightenment to the latter part of the twentieth century – the realm of 'self' tended to be off limits to medicine, which took as its object of enquiry the organic, physical body. The logic of this focus lay in the rationalism of the scientific method, which must, by definition, set aside factors that cannot be quantified and categorized in objective terms. Setting them aside, though, is not the same as dismissing them, as critics of biomedicine tend to imply. On the contrary; it is the moral authority of the free-willing individual that endorses the expertise of the medical practitioner.

At the heart of this 'classical' medical exchange is a division of labour in which medical science attends to the body of man to the extent that the body of man is thought to compromise his will. This is the nub of the Cartesian view of health, which stands in direct contrast to the non-Cartesian view, which presumes an understanding of health as a quality already written in nature, with which we should co-exist, rather than continually struggle. The tensions inherent in the modern human condition, between our animal past and our human future – between essence and existence, if you will – are themselves posed as the problem.

And, as we have seen, this tension is also the root of free will and the impetus to transcend nature's agenda and create our own. To live on, out and beyond immediate organic circumstance is a hallmark of human consciousness that we tend to take for granted. It underwrites our capacity to think of ourselves as autonomous individuals. But the implication of this is an obligation to daily affirm our freedom, both externally, in relation to a wider social world, and also internally, in relation to our own organic selves. 'Whatever is to be reckoned among the specific endowments of human nature does not lie in back of human freedom but in its domain, which every single individual must always take possession of anew if he would be a man', wrote Helmuth Plessner (1892–1985), who grasped so well the tension between *being* and *having* a body.[70] To 'have freedom of decision regarding different alternatives', wrote the brilliant psychologist Kurt Goldstein (1878–1965) 'is a characteristic peculiarity of man'. Recognising this 'peculiarity' is the key, said Goldstein, to unlocking the meaning of disease in man – as interruption of 'his necessity to realize his nature by free decision'.[71] 'We "have with us,"' wrote Maurice Merleau-Ponty (1908–1961), 'all that we need to transcend ourselves … choice and action alone cut us loose from our anchorage'.[72]

49

The freedom to choose and act is also the freedom to *not choose* and *not act*. Should the 'whips and scorns of time' seem too much, a retreat from temporal existence can seem attractive: to 'end the heart ache and the thousand natural shocks that flesh is heir to' might seem, in ones darker moments, 'a consummation devoutly to be wished'.[73] In the main, though, we choose life. And in choosing life we deny death, with the active support and assistance of modern scientific medicine. Life and death are the ultimate duality, of which man – and man alone – is most acutely conscious. There is no death in nature, only blind evolutionary force driving the life of a bacterium as much as a Bonobo. But for Enlightenment man there is something unique about human life that cannot be reduced to organic origins. That transcendental 'something' has often been understood in religious terms. But in the main it amounts to an entirely secular capacity, what Plessner terms 'a sustaining conception, that of being human – self-determining, responsible'[74] – freedom, in other words. Knowing what this means though, is a political question that has become deeply confused in the twentieth century.

Conclusion

The sad story of Albert Alexander, a 43-year-old policeman who scratched his face on a rose bush in 1941 is an apposite example to end with. The wound turned septic and his condition rapidly deteriorated. 'In great pain, desperately and pathetically ill' he was started on penicillin, then in its very earliest stages of development. 'But on the fifth day ... the supply of penicillin was exhausted. Inevitably, his condition deteriorated and he died a month later'. A terrible fate for Albert Alexander, his death nonetheless, writes James Le Fanu, 'has a metaphorical significance – a reminder to future generations of the crucial transitional moment between human susceptibility to the purposeless malevolence of bacteria and the ability, thanks to science, to defeat it'.[75]

In vanquishing 'the purposeless malevolence of bacteria' scientific medicine acts as an instrument of man's purposeful ambition. Nature is bent to serve the interests of that most unnatural of categories – man. But this is not an inevitable or one-way development. It hinges upon an active and questing sense of self-interest at the widest, social level, where the discipline of medical science must ultimately be legitimated. Without that endorsement even the boldest and most innovative of biomedical methods and discoveries struggle to win acceptance, and trust falls away.

Discussion topics

- Are the greatest achievements of modern medicine a product of the Cartesian dualist legacy, and if so, why?
- Explain what 'holism' is; what are the benefits and disadvantages of applying this approach to medicine?
- Which historical and cultural factors might account for the decline of the Cartesian dualist approach to medicine?

Further reading

Gay, P. (1967) The Enlightenment as medicine and as cure. In W.H. Barber, J.H. Brumfitt, R.A. Leigh, R. Shackleton, and S.S.B. Taylor (eds), *The Age of Enlightenment: Studies Presented to Theodore Besterman.* London: Oliver and Boyd.

A fine, pithy celebration of the primacy of medical knowledge and practice within the overall discourse of Enlightenment. Should this be hard to trace, Volume II of Peter Gay (1969) *The Enlightenment: An Interpretation* is on 'the science of freedom', and no less informative.

Greco, M. (1993) Psychosomatic subjects and the 'duty to be well': personal agency within medical rationality. *Economy and Society,* 22(3): 357–72.

Greco considers how one branch of modern medicine (psychosomatics) does indeed attend to subjective/biographical experience, but tends thereby to construct pathology in terms of disordered lifestyle. In contrast to Kleinman, Greco interrogates the consequences of a medical paradigm that goes beyond the body.

Kleinman, A. (1993) What is Specific to Western Medicine? In W.F. Bynum and R. Porter (eds), *Companion Encyclopedia of the History of Medicine.* London: Routledge.

Kleinman is critical of biomedicine for its narrow focus upon objectively verifiable pathology at the expense of subjectively experienced suffering. His anthropological approach usefully lays bare some of the underlying assumptions of twentieth-century medical practice in the West.

References

1 Irvine, D. (2000) 'Update on revalidation' *Journal of the Royal College of Physicians,* 34: 5415–17. On the Inquiry see Kennedy, I. (2001) Learning from Bristol: The Report of the Public Inquiry into Children's Heart Surgery at the Bristol Royal Infirmary 1984–1995. *Bristol Royal Infirmary Inquiry.* London, p. 530.
2 Royal Liverpool Children's Inquiry (2001) London: House of Commons.
3 See the Brian Deer website at http://briandeer.com/wakefield/legal-aid.htm. Take-up of the triple jab for two-year-olds declined from 92% in the mid-1990s, to 81% in 2004–5. In 2005–6 it rose to 84%. Data from The Information Centre for Health and Social Care, at http://www.ic.nhs.uk/
4 Smith, R. (2001) 'Why are doctors so unhappy.' *British Medical Journal,* 322: 1073–4.
5 Turnberg, L. (2000) 'Science, Society and the Perplexed Physician' *Journal of the Royal College of Physicians,* 34: 6569–75.
6 Jones, R. (2002) 'Declining Attruism' *British Medical Journal,* 324: 624–5.
7 Department of Health 'NHS R&D Programme : Research on the role of complementary and alternative medicine (CAM) in the care of patients with cancer'.
8 Smallwood, C. (2005) The role of complementary and alternative medicine in the NHS: an investigation into the potential contribution of mainstream complementary therapies to healthcare in the UK. Freshminds. London, p. 194,

p. 21. See also Select Committee on Science and Technology Sixth Report (2000). Ch.1.14ff 'Growing Use of CAM in the United Kingdom'.

9   Norwich Union, 'Health of the Nation Index 6'.

10 Tovey, P., Easthope, G. and Adams, J. (eds) (2003) *The Mainstreaming of Complementary and Alternative Medicine: Studies in Social Context.* London: Routledge. Kelner, M., Wellmana, B., Welsha, S. and Boona, H. (2006) 'How far can complementary and alternative medicine go? The case of chiropractic homeopathy'. *Social Science & Medicine,* 63 (10): 2617–27.

11 'Over the past decade, several British universities have started offering bachelor of science (BSc) degrees in alternative medicine, including six that offer BSc degrees in homeopathy'. Giles, J. (2007) 'Degrees of homeopathy stated as unscientific' *Nature,* 446: 352–3.

12 Homeopathic Hospitals are in London, Bristol, Glasgow, Liverpool and Tunbridge Wells, Kent.

13 See The NHS Directory of Complementary and Alternative Practitioners at http://www.nhsdirectory.org/

14 Atwell, B.L. (2003) 'Mainstreaming complementary and alternative medicine in the face of uncertainty' *UMKC Law Review,* 72: 3593–630.

15 Kleinman, A. (1993) In W.F. Bynum and R. Porter (eds), *Companion Encyclopedia of the History of Medicine,* Vol. 1 London: Routledge, p. 19.

16 Tarnas, R. (1996) *The Passion of the Western Mind: Understanding the Ideas That Have Shaped Our World View.* London: Pimlico, p. 303.

17 Trilling, L. (1972) *Sincerity and Authenticity.* Oxford: Oxford University Press, p. 24.

18 Sennett, R. (1986) *The Fall of Public Man.* London: Faber & Faber, p. 22.

19 Bookchin, M. (1995) *Re-enchanting Humanity: A Defense of the Human Spirit Against Anti-humanism, Misanthropy, Mysticism and Primitivism.* London: Cassell, p. 250.

20 Miller, J. (1978) *The Body in Question.* London: Jonathan Cape, p. 56.

21 Berger, P.L. (1971) *The Social Construction of Reality: A Treatise in the Sociology of Knowledge.* Harmondsworth: Penguin, p. 174.

22 Miller, J. (1978) ibid., p. 85.

23 Gillott, J. and Kumar, M. (1995) *Science and the Retreat from Reason.* London: Merlin Press, p. 137.

24 Le Fanu, J. (2000) *The Rise and Fall of Modern Medicine.* London: Abacus, p. 185–6. Barry Marshall and Robin Warren were awarded the Nobel Prize in 2005 for having discovered 'the bacterium Helicobacter pylori and its role in gastritis and peptic ulcer disease'.

25 See Maxeiner, D. and Miersch, M. (2006) In J. Panton and O.M. Hartwich (eds), *Science vs Superstition: The Case For a New Scientific Enlightenment.* London: Policy Exchange.

26 House of Lords Select Committee on Science and Technology: Sixth Report (2000).

27 ibid. Ch. 2: Disciplines examined: Definitions of the Various CAM Therapies, 2.14.

28 Kleinman, A. (1993) ibid., p. 18.

29 House of Lords Select Committee on Science and Technology: Sixth Report (2000): 2.15.

30 Professor Edzard Ernst, Professor in Complementary Medicine at Exeter University, in his submission to the Select Committee Report, at 1.12.

31 Descartes, R. (1637) In E. Chavez-Arvizo (ed.) (1997), *Descartes: Key Philosophical Writings.* London: Wordsworth Editions, pp. 71–122.

32 On engagement in and disengagement from nature, and its relationship to subjectivity, see Taylor, C. (1989) *Sources of the Self: The Making of Modern Identity*. Cambridge, MA: Harvard.

33 Iago to Roderigo in *Othello*: 'If the balance of our lives had not one scale of reason to poise another of sensuality, the blood and baseness of our natures would conduct us to most preposterous conclusions: but we have reason to cool our raging motions, our carnal stings, our unbitted lusts' (Act I; Scene II).

34 Locke, J. (1690) *An Essay Concerning Human Understanding*. Book II, Chapter XXI Of Power Para: 48.

35 Kleinman, A. (1993) ibid., p. 18.

36 Carter, R.B. (1983) *Descartes' Medical Philosophy: The Organic Solution to the Mind–Body Problem*. Baltimore, MD: Johns Hopkins University Press, p. 128.

37 Dollery, C. (1978) *The End of an Age of Optimism: Medical Science in Retrospect and Prospect*. London: Nuffield Provincial Hospitals Trust, p. 87.

38 Gay, P. (1967) In W.H. Barber, J.H. Brumfitt, R.A. Leigh, R. Shackleton and S.S. Taylor (eds), *The Age of Enlightenment: Studies Presented to Theodore Besterman*. Edinburgh: Oliver and Boyd, p. 380.

39 Porter, R. (1999) *The Greatest Benefit to Mankind: A Medical History of Humanity from Antiquity to the Present*. London: Fontana Press, p. 302.

40 Gay, P. (1969) *The Enlightenment: An Interpretation: Vol. II: The Science of Freedom*. London: Weidenfeld & Nicholson, p. 12.

41 Gross, P. R. and Levitt, N. (1994) *Higher Superstition: The Academic Left and Its Quarrels with Science*. Baltimore, MD: Johns Hopkins University Press, p. 20.

42 Bellow, S. (1965) *Herzog*. Harmondsworth: Penguin, p. 135.

43 See Rothman, D.J. (2003) *Strangers at the Bedside: A History of How Law and Bioethics Transformed Medical Decision Making*. New York: Aldine de Gruyter. (Ch.3 'The Gilded Age of Research').

44 Kleinman, A. (1993) ibid., p. 21.

45 Gross, P.R. and Levitt, N. (1994) ibid., p. 24.

46 Bloom, W. (ed.) (2000) *Holistic Revolution: The Essential New Age Reader*. London: Allen Lane/The Penguin Press, p. 149.

47 Arney, W.R. and Bergen, B.J. (1984) *Medicine and the Management of Living: Taming the Last Great Beast*. Chicago: University of Chicago Press, p. 2.

48 Select Committee on Science and Technology Third Report (Chapter 2: 'Public Attitudes and values,' 2.65).

49 Reith Lecture 2000: Respect for the Earth. Lecture No. 6 'A Royal View ...'.

50 See the excellent book by Alster, K.B. (1989) *The Holistic Health Movement*. Tuscaloosa, AL: University of Alabama Press. See also Sullivan, M. (2003) 'The new subjective medicine: taking the patient's point of view on health care and health'. *Social Science and Medicine*, 56: 1595–1604 and Greco, M. (1993) 'Psychosomatic subjects and "the duty to be well": personal agency within medical rationality'. *Economy and Society*, 22: 357–72.

51 A classic statement here is that of Goldstein, K. (1939) *The Organism: A Holistic Approach to Biology, Derived from Pathological Data in Man*. New York: American Book Company. See also the reference to Berger, P.L. (1971) ibid.

52 Porter, R. (1993) ibid. See also Sointu, E. (2006) 'The search for wellbeing in alternative and complementary health practices' *Sociology of Health & Illness*, 28: 3330–49.

53 See Carey, B. (2007) In *The New York Times* on how brain injury is said to affect moral choices (22 March, 2007).

54 Henig, R.M. ibid., Rose, S. (2005) 'Human agency in the neurocentric age' *EMBO reports,* 6 (11): 1001–5. Pinker, S. (2007) 'The mystery of consciousness' in *Time* 19th January.

55 de Waal, F. (1997) *Good Natured: Origins of Right and Wrong in Humans and Other Animals.* Cambridge, MA: Harvard University Press and Carey, B. (2007) ibid.

56 See de Waal, F. (2006) *Primates and Philosophers: How Morality Evolved.* Princeton, NJ: Princeton University Press.

57 Malik, K. (2000) *Man, Beast and Zombie: What Science Can and Cannot Tell Us About Human Nature.* London: Weidenfeld & Nicholson, p. 363.

58 See Goldstein, K. (1939) *The Organism: A Holistic Approach to Biology, Derived from Pathological Data in Man.* New York: American Book Company. See also Canguilhem, G. (1966) *On the Normal and the Pathological.* Dordrecht: D. Reidel and Plessner, H.K. (1970) *Laughing and Crying: A Study of the Limits of Human Behaviour.* Evanston, IL.: Northwestern University Press.

59 Lovelock, J. (1979) *Gaia: A New Look at Life on Earth.* Oxford: Oxford University Press.

60 Sharpe, M. and Wessely, S. (1997) 'Non-specific ill health: a mind-body approach to functional somatic symptoms' in A. Watkins (ed.), *Mind–Body Medicine: A Clinician's Guide to Psychoneuroimmunology.* New York: Churchill Livingston, p. 171.

61 An excellent introduction to this area is Morris, D. B. (1997) 'Placebo, Pain and Benefit: A Biocultural Model' in A. Harrington (ed.), *The Placebo Effect: An Interdisciplinary Exploration.* Cambridge, MA: Harvard University Press and also Moerman, D. (2002) *Meaning, Medicine, and the 'Placebo Effect'.* Cambridge: Cambridge University Press.

62 See, inter alia, Berger, J. (1967) *A Fortunate Man.* London: Writers and Readers. Selzer, R. (1982) *Letters to a Young Doctor.* New York: Touchstone and various works by A. Chekhov and L. Tolstoy.

63 For the classic formulation of the sick role as the central organising principle of the doctor–patient relationship, see Parsons, T. (1951) *The Social System.* London: Routledge & Kegan Paul.

64 Royal College of Physicians (2005) *Doctors in Society: Medical Professionalism in a Changing World.* Report of a Working Party of the Royal College of Physicians. London: Royal College of Physicians, p. 54.

65 Gaskell, G., Einsiedel, E., Hallman, W. Priest, S.H., Jackson, J. and Olsthoorn, J. (2005) 'Social values and the governance of science' *Science,* 310: 1908–9.

66 Singh, J., Hallmayer, J. and Illes, J. (2007) 'Interacting and paradoxical forces in neuro science and society' *Nature Reviews Neuroscience,* 8: 2153–60. p. 159.

67 Harrington, A. (1996) *Reenchanted Science: Holism in German Culture from Wulhelm II to Hitler.* Princeton, NJ: Princeton University Press; Rosenberg, C.E. (1998) Holism in Twentieth-Century Medicine in C. Lawrence and G. Weisz (eds), *Greater than the Parts: Holism in Biomedicine, 1920–1950.* New York, NY: Osford University Press. See also Jay, M. (1984) *Marxism and Totality: The Adventures of a Concept from Lukacs to Habermas.* London: Polity, who makes the point that holism is as much a concept of the left as it is of the right.

68 Lawrence, C. and Weisz, G. (eds) (1998) 'Medical holism: the context' in *Greater Than the Parts: Holism in Biomedicine, 1920–1950.* New York: Oxford University Press, p. 2.

69 See Alster, K.B. (1989) ibid., p. 83.

70 Plessner, H.K. (1970) ibid., p. 10. See also Berger, P. L. (1971) ibid. on the 'continuing internal dialectic between identity and its biological substratum. The

individual continues to experience himself as an organism, apart from and sometimes set against the socially derived objectifications of himself. Often this dialectic is apprehended as a struggle between a "higher" and a "lower" self, respectively equated with social identity and pre-social, possibly anti-social animality. The higher self must repeatedly assert itself over the "lower", sometimes in critical tests of strength' (pp. 203–4).

71 Goldstein, K. (1939) ibid., 450.
72 Merleau-Ponty, M. (1962) *Phenomenology of Perception*. London: Routledge, p. 456.
73 *Hamlet* Act 3, Scene 1.
74 Plessner, H.K. (1970) ibid., p. 10.
75 Le Fanu, J. (2000) ibid., p. 6.

4

Health Scares and Risk Awareness

Adam Burgess

- The prevalence of health scares suggests a profound shift in the way we think about the world.
- The 'risk society' is a very recent and specific development.
- Risk awareness has become a new moral code bound up with mistrust, withdrawal from social interaction and the formalising of informal life.
- Scares cannot be understood by their 'scary' characteristics alone; we also have to understand the wider social context and background.
- Alarms are created by particular actors and institutions and can flourish given the defensiveness of scientific and political authority.

Try to read a newspaper or news magazine, listen to radio, or watch television; on any day some alarm bells will be ringing. What are Americans afraid of? Nothing much, really, except the food they eat, the water they drink, the air they breathe, the land they live on, and the energy they use. In the amazingly short time of fifteen to twenty years, confidence about the physical world has turned into doubt. Once the source of safety, science and technology have become the source of risk.
Mary Douglas and Aaron Wildavsky, *Risk and Culture*, 1982.

The risk society

In modern western societies health-related scares and alarms have become routine. There are countless 'risky' problems drawn to our attention by the media and government, and we appear to have become more receptive to worrying about them. This trend emerged first in the United States in the late 1960s and early 1970s, as the above quotation from one of the more important books on risk suggests.[1] More recently in the UK and Europe, we have become accustomed to sudden revelations that foods we eat and everyday technologies we use may actually be harming us. Archetypal is the story suggesting that something hitherto assumed to be inconsequential, even pleasurable, such as eating meat, using deodorant or a mobile phone, has been discovered to be *associated with* an above-average incidence of a particular complaint. Even when research is dismissed by the majority of scientists – as in the case of the study claiming an association between the MMR vaccine and autism – conflicting views among apparent experts may be enough to confirm for many people the possibility of a threat, and suggest we take precautionary measures by steering clear of the subject of controversy.

Our apparent susceptibility to often rather obscure alarms is more ironic than is often recognised. We are surely more worldly and 'knowing' than ever – captured by the remarkable ease with which we deal with and absorb new technologies into our lives. By contrast, even relatively recently, a general lack of familiarity with science and technology sometimes combined with established superstitions to ridiculous effect. It was widely believed that the speed of early rail travel would cause injury, as the human body simply was not designed to manage such velocity. To an extent, such attitudes were associated with an older generation less familiar with and open to innovation. Thus a well-known cartoon pictures an elderly lady staring up at a light socket (we assume shortly after the introduction of electricity to her home), without a bulb with the thought bubble that perhaps 'electricity was leaking all over the house'.[2]

Despite greater freedom from traditional dogma and more familiarity with technology, alarms about improbable dangers sometimes make more of an impact on society than ever before. During an earlier period of 'classical modernity' in the nineteenth and early twentieth centuries, society was often more open to the spirit of experimentation; the very opposite of the contemporary culture of risk and anxiety. Even if it was believed by some in the past that train travel might be dangerous, these feelings were not allowed to get in the way of progress. Risk was balanced against benefits, and typically found to be a more acceptable 'price to be paid' than is now the norm. Today, an influential mode of thought suggests that because we have 'played God' by 'meddling with nature' through techniques of genetic engineering, for example, that some kind of natural order has been disrupted and there will be an inevitable, if unknown price to pay. The metaphor of Frankenstein's monster is often invoked by the media and captures this sense of a revenge of nature. The term, 'Frankenfoods' was used to describe genetically modified foodstuffs, for example, and approvingly described by a prominent environmentalist as, 'a stroke of instinctive tabloid genius'.[3] In a more elaborate form, the original thesis that we live in a 'risk society' suggested that we are now paying the environmental price for the unthinking process of modernization that created the industrial world.[4] Closer scrutiny of the subject of such fears reveals a pattern of them having little foundation, however. It is unclear in what terms crops that have been subject to genetic rather than more traditional modification might pose a human health hazard, for example. There may be a hypothetical hazard from electromagnetic fields generated by a mobile phone as opposed to the plainly ridiculous idea of 'leaking' electricity, but in real human terms there sometimes seems little to distinguish the old and new forms of technological risk aversion. In a sense we do not seem to have made much advance on the old lady's misunderstanding of electricity – and at least she had the excuse of dealing with the new and unknown.

Technology as threat

Part of the explanation for our sometimes increased suspicion of technology is that since the turn of the twentieth century humanity has been struck by a series of profoundly negative experiences, most notably two world wars, that have tempered our previous optimism. The world's experience of devastation from nuclear weapons and a series of near misses at power plants have created suspicion rather than enthusiasm for 'radiation'. Yet we can also see that there is little direct relationship between these negative experiences and the extreme caution that is now exercised. The contrast between the actually quite limited human impact of the Chernobyl nuclear accident and the mass devastation it was assumed to have caused suggests we have come to expect the very worst irrespective of the evidence, for example.[5] There has been no directly related tragic incident that explains why we should be so anxious about genetic technology or the use of microwaves in communication. Mistrust and suspicion appear to have taken on a life of their own, and aspects of our lives now revolve around keeping such risks at bay – from eating organic foods and avoiding pesticides, to guarding our drinks in nightclubs in case they are 'spiked' by a mysterious stranger.

Do these scares and alarms really matter? After all, many of them strike us as plain silly, and what damage can be done by imagining more 'pure' products will keep risk at bay? In some cases it is clear that alarms are of concern, as they have manifestly negative consequences. The MMR scare has led to a serious fall in vaccination rates in the UK, raising the spectre of more children contracting the diseases against which it protects: measles, mumps and rubella.[6] Measles is a potentially fatal disease, highlighting the irony that some parents find themselves exposing their children to a proven deadly risk because of concern over a disproved one. Risk anxieties can be particularly fraught in such cases of *competing risk* where insulation against one risk, exposes one to another (larger) one. In other cases there seem to be no consequences to health alarms, as in the case of the constant warnings about radiation from mobile phones promoted by the British media from the late 1990s. The importance of mobile phones in our lives has led us to, ultimately, ignore these health concerns. This example illustrates how, to some extent, our avoidance of risk is governed by the availability of choice; there is no ready alternative to the mobile phone, whereas we can relatively easily avoid GM foods – and even go for the organic alternative.

Reactions to health risk alarms are rarely straightforward. There is sometimes a process we can describe as *risk migration*, where the focus of anxiety is subject to change.[7] While we ultimately chose to continue using mobile phones themselves, many people seemed to have shifted their concerns onto a different part of the same technology that seems less immediately necessary. People continue to campaign against mobile phone masts, despite the fact that human harm from these structures is even more scientifically implausible than from handsets. It is not unusual for risk concerns to make only a short-term impact, such as in the case of the GM food alarm that subsided by the middle of the first decade of the twenty-first century. And who now recalls the 'millennium bug' that was going to devastate the world's computer systems?[8] The passing of one concern does not seem to prevent new concerns appearing to effectively 'take the place' of the last alleged threat to our health, however.

While the public has 'bought in to' particular health scares and alarms to very varying degrees, it is clear that we do not believe everything we read. This should be recalled when we find ourselves so readily blaming the media for the latest scare. The media are generally only able to influence the general terms in which we think about risks.[9] The detail of stories is rarely recalled, suggesting the influence of the media is indirect. It is also possible to detect an explicit cynicism about health scares, particularly in the UK where they have become such a staple of 'news' reporting.

Since the health scare about salmonella in eggs in 1988, the British public have been inundated with media health alarms and it is unsurprising that many people have grown (selectively) sceptical. Consider this response from a member of the public to the first phase of scares about 'mad cow disease' back in 1992:

It's a lot of nonsense really. I mean, to think that the government would allow us to be put at risk from such a thing is ridiculous. The media are just playing things up again and trying to scare us. I don't believe a word of it, and I certainly haven't stopped eating meat.[10]

There are clearly limits to any assumption of public gullibility about the media and risks. Impact also depends upon the extent of opportunity to influence the terms of discussion – an extent that is limited in cases such as the outbreak of the disease SARS which appeared from nowhere and was relatively quickly resolved in 2003.[11] It should be added that the limits of media influence are not for the want of them trying to make the news, rather than just report it. Especially in the UK, and illustrated by examples such as mobile phones and GM foods, particular newspapers and television programmes have set out to consciously campaign against particular technologies, and for particular risks. While the *Daily Mail* newspaper is most notoriously associated with this approach, it is by no means confined to this newspaper or indeed more populist 'tabloid' newspapers in general. In the case of mobile phone fears 'quality' outlets like the *BBC* and *The Times* were central to the construction of alarm.[12]

Risk perceptions and the reorganisation of life

Thinking more widely and sociologically, it is not the extent to which we firmly believe in a particular scare that is most significant. Nor is it necessarily the actual threat said to be posed that is of lasting importance. One of the striking characteristics of contemporary health alarms is that the majority are so quickly forgotten, suggesting the purported threat was minor, illusory or simply one about which little more could meaningfully be said or done. It is the individual and cumulative social *response* to health threats and alarms that is likely to be more consequential, irrespective of the threat itself. Recall that it has long been understood that panic can be a bigger problem than its ostensible source. There were large-scale deaths in theatres in the late nineteenth/early twentieth century, for example. These were as likely to be brought about by crushing that followed a false alarm, as they were by the effects of real fire. This, perhaps curious phenomenon, is expressed by the increasing importance accorded *perceptions of risk*, as opposed to the actual *objective risk* posed, and is at the heart of the social study of risk.[13] Thus it is widely accepted that scientifically there is no evidence that the radiation emitted by mobile phone masts can cause human harm. Nonetheless, policy initiatives such as the official British inquiry into the issue insisted that people's perceptions that there *might be* became central to how the issue was handled. In an age where authority is anxious to be seen to be taking public health seriously, it is felt that even such suspicions must be somehow acknowledged, even if it is difficult to actually do anything about them. This was reflected in the conduct and findings of the official inquiry into the issue which was anxious to entertain anything apparently related to public concern.[14]

Risk perceptions have apparently taken on a life of their own, freed from the restrictions of more scientific or objective assessment. There are other ways in which unfounded claims of potential harm gain authority, and reasons why these might make an impact irrespective of real confirmation. Until relatively recently it was thought to be the job of politicians, scientists and health officials to alert us only in case of a clear threat to the population at large and when practical steps necessary to containment were deemed necessary. In modern Britain, since the experiences of handling AIDS and BSE/vCJD in the 1980s, by contrast, it has become routine for authorities to publicly share their own worst-case scenarios. This was the case with dramatic predictions of large-scale casualties from bird flu in late 2005, for example, despite the significant barriers to it becoming a serious human health problem. It was a case of 'when, not if' we faced a deadly flu epidemic, according to the government's chief medical officer.[15] In the past such claims might have been dismissed as irresponsible scaremongering, given that there was no clear purpose or benefit to such action other than exonerating the authorities from any subsequent accusation of a failure to forewarn. In a society that has become culturally risk-averse, however, such messages can strike a chord with personal insecurity and the strongly held conviction that it is 'better to be safe than sorry'. Although these impacts depend on context and rarely endure, we can say that in the negotiation of risk *evidence has become relatively irrelevant compared to perceptions of risk*.

We are often urged to be 'aware' of risks no matter how rare the threat may be, or how difficult to identify. Self-monitoring for signs of certain diseases is recommended, for example, even though conclusive early diagnosis is difficult even for medical professionals. A striking feature of contemporary risk awareness is that it does not principally require or invite us to be, or become more factually informed. The emphasis is rather on demonstrating that we are somehow conscious of the problem and, better still, taking steps to simply avoid any kind of exposure. As we habitually *'think twice'* about what we expose ourselves to or digest, however, it is curiously uncertain what we actually *think about* other than avoiding what we might – sometimes very vaguely – recall being associated with a problem. For all the publicity about mobile phone masts over the last decade, for example, most people remain unclear about what the problem might be. In the absence of knowledge it is easy to fall back upon intuition about what 'seems to be right'; in recent times perhaps the most influential is the rejection of anything deemed 'unnatural'. Yet any strict division between the 'natural' and 'unnatural' is scientifically meaningless; there are no 'natural' or 'unnatural' chemicals, for example, only chemicals.[16] Nor is there any basis to the assumption that the more 'natural' must be better for us – sometimes quite the opposite, as products that have been subject to more direct human intervention and control may be safer. The meaning of the 'E numbers' that are so readily avoided when scouring product ingredients is simply that they have been rigorously tested for human consumption – unlike organic foods!

Regardless of its curiosities, 'healthy living' has become a mantra of our age, from government campaign, to supermarket slogan and personal credo. As the notion suggests, what we eat or are exposed to has taken on more significance than simple nourishment or pleasure, to instead say something about who we are and what we stand for. 'What's in your shopping basket?', ask magazine features, as they assess the healthiness of a celebrity's weekly food consumption, and thereby determine their virtue as an individual and role model. Living healthily and minimising risk has become part of many people's way of life; it is a conscious ritual pursued through abstinence from unhealthy (but secretly desirable!) commodities.[17]

It can be argued that risk awareness has become a new moral code through which we conduct our lives; despite the often very scientific, at least mathematical appearance of risk calculation it has a clear relationship to contemporary morality.[18] In one of the most important and influential books in this area, *Risk and Culture*,[19] the role and function that risk perceptions can acquire in cohering both more traditional, and modern American society was examined. The boundary between what is claimed to be 'natural' and 'unnatural' forms an enduring focus for what society deems acceptable, telling us what sort of society it really is, or aspires to be. From such a perspective, risk perceptions can be understood to perform a function for society comparable to religion or traditional morality. 'Awareness' of risks to our health and security has become *a new form of showing oneself to be a responsible citizen*; taking active measures to limit the impact of these evils an even greater sign of modern virtue.

In the past we were implored to avoid or abstain from what was deemed sinful by religious authority. Adultery and gluttony were precluded, for example, and their avoidance increased the chances of an afterlife free of torment. Yet we now live in an age where traditional moral prescriptions to avoid sin have little purchase; as traditional values have declined, even basic right and wrong are now unclear.[20] Contemporary western culture is characterised by confusion about what to do for the best, even though it still feels the need to make such distinctions. Aspects of a new secular morality to partially fill the vacuum left by traditional morality's decline can be discerned in the way that health and risk avoidance is promoted and negotiated. Drugs are no longer rejected in British society on the grounds that they are illegal or simply wrong, for example, but on the basis of the (relative) health risks with which they are associated.[21]

It is not only in relation to our own health that elements of a new moral code can be identified. As the example of the MMR vaccine indicates, we are at our most vulnerable when considering risks to our children. Although many parents are aware that the threat of 'stranger danger' is remote, and the risks to a child's wellbeing from 'wrapping them in cotton wool' are considerable, the responsible parent is now one who demonstrates extreme caution with regard to their child's movement and whereabouts.[22] The fear of attack from 'stranger danger' appears now to be of greater concern than the potential for accidental injuries. Outdoor play and independent activity are now policed and curtailed as the pattern of family life has changed. It is in this realm that the ultimate logic of heightened risk perception – the basic *withdrawal from social activity* is clearest. In its own terms life, particularly young life, is one big risk and increased withdrawal from engagement with it is the only certain path to safety. Yet this is not to suggest that young people are all now imprisoned in their own homes. What it does mean is that exposure to the outside world tends to be more self-conscious, regulated and monitored – through the use of mobile phones, for example.[23]

There are two other related consequences that the elevation of risk perception is having on society. Related to increased social withdrawal is an *increase in mistrust*, a widely recognised malaise of late modern society.[24] Sometimes explicitly, at other times only implicitly, risk awareness preaches vigilance that is particularly directed towards the unknown. The message of drug-assisted 'date rape' awareness in universities is to 'trust nobody', for example. Any male could be trying to add 'roofies' to your drink, so attention is required as well as a device to protect your drink, according to what has been described as a 'synthetic panic'.[25] The questioning of any unfamiliar face near events and activities involving children such as football clubs in modern

Britain is likely to invite even greater mistrust and hostility, irrespective of any relationship to incidents that have actually taken place in such settings.

A related development is that the erosion of trust involves the closing-down of informal, unregulated space, or what we might describe as the *formalising of the informal*.[26] While informal interaction must continue in our society, the logic of risk awareness is that the relationship be subject to contract and formal, even external scrutiny, and this transforms the character of social experience. Thus formally innocent informal activities, such as photographing one's children taking part in school events, often now require formalised consent. Now a suspicious activity, the photographing of children in public space becomes a self-conscious act subject to the approval of authority – instead of capturing moments of human joy. The comfort and help of children by carers and teachers have become more difficult as any form of physical touching of children has become problematic.[27]

The emergence and understanding of modern risk

Particularly for those too young to have experienced society before the 1980s, it may be difficult to appreciate the novelty of a life shaped by the negotiation of everyday risks. Even for older generations, the elevation of risks has now become routine. It can now be difficult to recall a very different, if relatively recent, world when food was principally a source of sustenance (and occasionally one of pleasure!), and childhood involved leaving home in the morning and returning only for supper, away from constant parental gaze – as was the case in this author's experience of adolescence in the 1970s.

Risk alarms about minor or hypothetical threats and heightened perceptions of risk separate from experience are generally particular to the modern, 'western' world. Still in contemporary Africa, people confront direct threats to their survival rather than the more remote and changing health anxieties with which we are familiar. The lack of clean water and basic medicines in many parts of the world even today mean that the prospect of serious illness and premature death continue to haunt those societies. Given such very real problems, it is difficult to imagine widespread social anxiety about more remote ones like mobile phone radiation. It is likely to strike those confronted by continual shortages of food as bizarre to worry about whether it was genetically modified, or produced by the more conventional process of human modification – agriculture. There is a geography of risk related to the extent to which basic needs have been satisfied, allowing a focus on less immediate concerns. By the same logic we can begin to appreciate that the perception of health risks is not just peculiar to modern times, but the very recent past. After all, it is only during the last century that even developed societies have been able to relatively easily sustain their populations, manage the main killer infectious diseases and find themselves in the luxurious position of being able to worry about what they (partially) choose.

Considering risk involves calculating the impact of our own actions rather than accepting fate. This is illustrated by the important *distinction between a risk and a hazard*. Hazard is the potential effect of a situation, process or product, such as it being unstable, corrosive or carcinogenic. Risk refers to the actual chance of something happening, taking account of real behaviour or exposure. This is often expressed as a probability. Everything we do exposes us to hazards, from knives in the kitchen to cars on the road. It is how we do things, and how often, that determines the risk. So, for instance, stairs are a hazard, but it is the likelihood of injury that is known as the risk. The latter will be a function of variables such as step height, lighting conditions, age and speed.

Forgetting current associations with threat and hazard for a moment, the concept of risk essentially concerns the idea of *probability*. Where there are seen to be different possible outcomes people can think about taking a risk; gambling on what may or may not happen. In this sense risk is also bound up with conceiving of *the future*, as these outcomes are not yet determined, and will only become clear with the passage of time. As sociologists and anthropologists have observed, the concept of risk did not exist in pre-modern societies.[28] It was not generally possible in these societies to realistically conceive of the future, and hence of probability. Instead, pre-modern societies were generally dominated by *the present* as a struggle for basic survival, and the past in terms of the legacy of ancestors and the word of God(s). In so far as they imagined the future it was likely to be the unearthly one of a possible afterlife. There was not widespread acceptance that things could happen purely by accident rather than being a sign of having pleased or displeased divine forces.[29]

This did not reflect a collective stupidity, so much as the conditions of life that they endured. Conceiving of different future outcomes suggests particular kinds of activity and a particular way of life. Traditional societies were typically dominated by a routine of agricultural subsistence, where new possibilities were slow to present themselves. Reflecting their generally more fragile existence at the mercy of nature, things happened *to them* rather than them being able to *make things happen* through their own planning and activity. The crops might inexplicably fail and the whole community be immediately threatened as a consequence. They could scarcely conceive of being able to control their lives in the present, let alone the future. Even in the early modern England of the seventeenth century it was generally understood that illness was fundamentally a judgement of God, and therefore little could realistically be done to cure the ailment – other than change one's (moral) ways.[30]

There are certainly moments in pre-modern societies where a sense of risk begins to emerge. Yet the concept of risk really only makes sense in the socio-economic system of capitalism which is essentially concerned with making profit, and has to take future-dependent risks to do so.[31] When people begin to systematically engage in trade and manufacturing certain products to sell on an (uncertain) market, people are taking risks whether they like it or not. And of course the market system remains with us today and the traditional sense of taking risks therefore retains an influence, even if in a more uncertain way than during capitalism's more confident early years. A qualification to the importance of the positive conception of risk in classical capitalism is that risk was rarely reflected upon as a distinct category; in the simplest sense *risks were what society took, rather than speculated about.*

A further historical distinction – in addition to that between pre-modern and modern – needs to be made between an earlier period of *classical modernity* up to the 1950s, and a subsequent *late modernity*. The *language of risk* was not nearly so common before the last few decades of the twentieth century but it was central to the *operation* of modern society as it emerged from the industrial, scientific and intellectual revolutions that ushered in the modern era. The difference was that risk prior to the 1960s/70s was generally understood in the more positive sense of *taking risks*, rather than the defensive sense of feeling *at risk*.[32]

While advanced modern societies faced what might broadly be termed negative risks before the 1960s, they were typically more remote, specific, and more within the realm of social and political influence. Thus the overriding international 'risk' in the decades following the Second World War was the threat of global nuclear war. To an extent, this produced mass panic and was an important fear in some people's lives, particularly in the United States. And of course, this was a 'risk' that threatened complete annihilation rather than the characteristically minor, even hypothetical risk of today. Nonetheless, the threat of nuclear war was understood to be contingent upon human, political activity – most importantly the state of relations between the then two 'superpowers', Russia and America. Pressure could be brought to bear on this relationship through mass campaigning activities to stop nuclear arms proliferation and insisting that their use was unacceptable. We can add that this was a distinctively global risk 'out there', rather than the everyday dangers woven into the fabric of our lives confronted today. Contemporary environmental risks, in particular, are fundamentally removed from the realm of human activity; the damage has been done according to this perspective and it is principally now a question of living with the consequences.[33]

It is only with the more personalised and pervasive sense of risk characteristic of the post-1960s period that it became the subject of intellectual investigation. Risk began to be thought about once these new risk perceptions became apparent and made an impact upon, first, American society. This is perhaps unsurprising; it is only once things become a problem that we typically set about trying to understand them. The context was that scientific, commercial and political authority in the USA was alarmed at an apparently sudden outburst of very public risk alarms in the late 1960s and early 1970s. Slightly earlier scares over cranberries, the pesticide DDT, and the sweetener saccharin, anticipated larger reactions over all manner of phenomena, as the quotation with which this chapter began indicates. The accumulation of scares suggested that Americans no longer trusted their businesses, scientists and government – to the extent that they would allow them to be poisoned by pesticides and even drinks sweeteners. Analysts were further struck by the apparent acceptance of some everyday real risks of some concern to experts, sometimes precisely among the people who became so animated about 'phantom' ones. These concerns and questions were reflected in the first article exploring contemporary risk, published in 1969.[34] The curious discrepancy between public and expert assessment of risk was central to this and subsequent accounts. Masses of articles and books on risk, mainly evolved from a psychological perspective, were produced and an industry of risk assessment and management began to flourish in its wake, drawing upon its tools and concepts.

So how did emerging experts attempt to understand growing risk concerns? This is a particularly relevant question given that the still growing industry of risk analysts and managers have not been clearly successful in encouraging the more balanced assessment of risk which it sought to do. In fact, an originally American condition has spread to the rest of the developed world, suggesting fundamental problems with their approach – assuming that analysis might be able to play a constructive role in moderating needless anxiety.

Studies of risk perception and the practice of risk management suggest that the reaction to particular risks can be indirectly 'read' from the characteristics of the object in question. The interaction between risk characteristics and individual psychology is the key to understanding (and potentially defusing) risk perceptions in the dominant paradigm.[35] A risk study might, for example, highlight how fear of flying may be improbable given the rarity of aircraft crashes, but nonetheless unsurprising given the unique 'dread' and apparent finality of a crash, and the lack of any sense of control for helpless passengers. Greater communication might be seen to alleviate helplessness; to help manage the risk. The amount of 'dread' that potential 'risk objects' inspire, how much apparent choice is involved, and how much control they appear to offer the subject, continue to be regarded as key predictors of a negative reaction. Combining the elements of hazard and risk, studies typically concentrate on exhaustive technical analyses of the potential hazard and risk, with experiments in how these are perceived.

The basic approach of risk studies has not fundamentally changed in its 35 year-odd history. The focus remains on the technical characteristics of, and psychological variables associated with risk objects. These are a useful introduction to understanding and can be interesting in their own right, yet have limited explanatory power. Take an example. It is useful to be aware of the characteristics of mobile phone radiation if one wants to set about understanding concerns, not least because it allows us to understand the scientific improbability of them having any harmful effect on humans. Further, considering factors such as whether a risk is chosen or imposed may help explain why some people are so angry about mobile phone masts (which they don't choose to be near), but not their handsets (which they do). Yet such factors fail to explain why such feelings vary so radically in intensity in different countries at different times; they do not explain why Italians appear to fear what they call 'electrosmog' so much more than people from Finland, for example. Why do most Americans appear happy to eat genetically modified food, while most Britons appear absolutely opposed? Psychological and science-based accounts simply cannot explain such differences.

Some of the problems associated with the basic concepts and assumptions of the technical/psychological approach to risk were usefully outlined by Douglas and Wildavsky (1982) who demonstrated the implausibility of clearly establishing distinctions such as between voluntary and involuntary risk in the real, social world. They indicated that reactions were bound up with their specific social and cultural context. The rise of environmentalism in American culture profoundly affected the perceptions of particular groups in their analysis, for example. The centrality of context can be illustrated by considering that even the most apparently clear-cut risk aversion is more conditional than it seems. Opposition to genetic experimentation is one of the most pronounced contemporary feelings, playing as it does upon a cultural script of the perils of 'playing God' and the horrors of the choices it might make available (Nazi inspired mythical 'designer babies'). In the language of risk communication and management it has a very high 'yuk' factor. Yet, as experiments inviting the public to taste a fictitious GM apple suggest, reactions are conditional upon context.[36] Asked a general question about GM foods in a survey, respondents are likely to demonstrate their awareness of a dominant message about healthy and responsible eating by rejecting them. However, given a more direct, actual choice curiosity may get the better of a largely imposed agenda about 'Frankenfoods'. Other research demonstrates the powerful influence of the media in 'framing' opinion and 'socially amplifying' issues related to GM foods.[37,38]

Studies of risk typically fail to take sufficient account of context and how that context is subject to continual change. Accounts have specifically failed to take account of how official reactions themselves are an important, sometimes defining part of the evolving issue. The way that authorities handled signs of growing but initially limited concern sometimes helps explain how some risk issues go on to become more significant, and others do not. The dismissal of any link between farmed salmon and ill health by the UK's Food Standards Agency meant that this American-inspired worry made no headway in Britain, for example. Since the first risk alarms in the 1960s the way that the authorities have responded is absolutely central to subsequent reactions, yet has remained of marginal interest to risk analysis. There has been some recognition that reactions can be inflamed by (apparently conspiratorial) silence from authorities; corporate failure to respond to damaging rumours is seen as unwise, for example.[39] Yet the now more common approach of authorities is not only to rarely challenge risk concerns but to advertise possible harms even before they become real. Such official pre-emptive warnings – such as was seen with mobile phones, bird flu and many others – are likely to trigger concern irrespective of knowledge about the object in question. Research on the impact of explanatory leaflets accompanying mobile phones found that far from allaying any concerns, in so far as any reaction could be discerned they stimulated it – on the basis that there must be something worth worrying about if the government thinks a warning is required.[40] The focus on the technical and psychological characteristics of risk has neglected not only other social and contextual factors in general, but specifically the determining role that signals of officialdom send out.

The technical and psychological emphasis has usefully been contested in recent sociological writings by for example, Beck[41] and Giddens.[42] At the same time, the sociological encounter with risk that they initiated tends to jump from the micro/psychological level of traditional risk studies to a grand macro-level of how general social forces have created risk perceptions. In such accounts it appears that risk is an inevitable product of the way in which society has developed in modern times. This takes no account of the role played by more intermediate developments, particular actors and a precise sense of what was happening in any given context. What is more, the tendency to 'objectify' the emergence of the risk society tends to objectify the risks themselves. While there are suggestions in the famous work of Beck that risks are created by social circumstance and particular actors, the overall emphasis is on the objectively given character of environmental risks and our powerlessness to even understand the threat, let alone contain it. Thus it was the particular and threatening qualities of radiation that were central to his account of the *Risk Society*, and its popularity (with its publication coming so soon after the Chernobyl nuclear accident). Yet it is clear that Beck knows little about the different forms of radiation, nor does he feel obliged to ground his assertions in scientific fact or empirical study. While the original 'risk society' thesis remains useful in emphasising what has changed about late modernity, it fails to clearly locate these changes in social rather than technical processes.

More usefully, approaches have evolved that aspire to focus on the social construction of risk, notably the now influential *social amplification of risk* framework.[43] To go further, however, requires separating out the different elements and actors at work in any given example. The most basic distinction to elaborate is between the general conditions that make risk alarms possible, and then the different actors and influences that determine which particular risk will become dominant.

Preconditions for the risk society

For the purposes of analysis and understanding, a distinction needs to be made between three different levels, from the broadest, macro-level, to the impact of intermediate factors, and then the specific role of particular institutions and actors. Taking account of all three elements can take us further in understanding why a particular society might be concerned with a particular risk at a particular time. We can first identify a set of factors that combine together to make a 'risk society', from the most fundamental to the more intangible.

Economic: 'post-material' society of consumer choice

As already suggested, the risk society is unimaginable where the basic necessities of life remain unavailable and most of our energy continues to be absorbed by the struggle for existence. A useful perspective here is the idea that we live in a 'post-material' world.[44] According to this theory, the increasing preoccupation with ideas such as environmentalism from which we do not stand to directly gain is understood as a luxury we can now afford. Having gone beyond the material stage, it is now possible for us to concern ourselves with ideas, choices ... and worries.

Medical: from specific causes to 'risk factors'

A significant change began to occur in how patterns of disease were identified from the mid-twentieth century that encouraged a new way of understanding modern ill health. Instead of identifying microbes as the sole and definite cause of disease, emphasis was increasingly placed on social, environmental and behavioural variables statistically *associated with* disease patterns. The turning point in the identification of *risks* (as opposed to distinct causes) came with the establishment of the association between cigarette smoking and numerous health problems in the 1950s and 1960s. Despite lacking the clear and specific causality traditionally associated with modern medicine (or an understanding of *how* disease was caused) the association between smoking and significant harm was declared definitive. Subsequently, far less statistically significant relationships than that between smoking and cancer have become sources of publicity, worry and dispute.

Scientific/technical: increased capacity to identify hazards

The risk society is unimaginable where we lack the capacity to identify hazards; conversely, the greater our capacity the greater is the potential for an increased number of risk concerns. Until society becomes aware of a link between smoking and lung cancer, for example, clearly the potential for alarm is restricted. Less obvious and much more problematic is the increasing number of examples involving the ability to identify theoretically harmful hazards in smaller and smaller quantities. Chemicals are a key example. We can now identify the presence of the tiniest amount of chemicals in our food and other products, and these discoveries have provided the basis for many recent risk alarms – and there are guaranteed to be more as the European Commission has launched its REACH initiative to investigate thousands of chemicals with 'proven or suspected hazardous properties'.[45] This is notwithstanding the fact that chemical danger always concerns their quantity, not inherently dangerous properties; in other words aspirin, for example, can be beneficial in small doses but harmful, even deadly, in larger quantities.

Structural/social: individualisation

The risk society is unimaginable where powerful collective institutions and habits dominate everyday life. A defining feature of modern societies is that they were also *mass* societies. We no longer lived in small isolated communities, and nor were we so susceptible to the suspicions and prejudices associated with such an existence. In the modern world our experiences were tempered by wider knowledge and associations that helped make sense of what might befall us. In the relatively recent past we were embedded in communities, political and recreational associations that created a feeling of collective confidence and wider responsibility. Even terrible experiences such as that of civilians during the bombing of London in the Second World War could be stoically endured, even celebrated. Being 'all in it together' makes for an entirely different experience of any misfortune. As is widely observed, late modern life is much more fragmented and disconnected from other institutions and associations; we rarely even watch the same television programmes today, or share in any kind of collective moments.[46] Experiencing life alone leaves us prey to greater uncertainty and doubt. The growth of a more individualistic human experience also directly suggests a preoccupation with personal health and survival. Disconnected from any wider sense of national or generational continuity, personal survival and longevity become paramount and leave us susceptible to a regime of risk awareness.

Cultural: end of deference

The risk society is unimaginable where the public accept lack of choice, and deference to traditional authority. Accompanying a society still shaped by need and lack of choice, attitudes were resigned to accept what was available regardless of any inherent risks or benefits. Britain was long distinguished by a reluctance to complain about goods and services, for example: with food rationing remaining in place until the 1950s and the relative absence of consumer goods there wasn't a lot of point! Intimately connected to deference is trust; people were also deferential because there was more unquestioning trust. Until the late modern period the medical opinion of doctors was rarely questioned, for example. Late modern society has developed both the ability to seek multiple sources of advice and the confidence to do so. This feeling is a powerful impulse creating openness to unknown, untold dangers. In response, authorities have become increasingly fearful of keeping anything from public scrutiny, even disclosure that in the past would have been called 'scaremongering'. This impulse is central to setting many contemporary risk alarms in motion.

Ideological: dystopian future

The risk society is unimaginable where society holds a firmly optimistic view of the future, and the benefits that human intervention and technology can bring. The assumption that human innovation must hold a potentially 'dark side' is particular to a world that has lost its faith in progress and the power of ideas to change the world.[47] Recall the example of the lack of concern about mobile phone radiation in Finland. Partly this is because, unusually, Finns to some degree retain a now old-fashioned view of the benefits of science and technology. Outside the context of confidence about human intervention and the future, change is likely to be experienced principally as threatening and a source of worry.

Political: end of politics and promotion of health

Closely related to the collapse of ideology is the end of politics in its classical modern form. The risk society is unimaginable where society is still shaped by competing visions of how society should be organised, and resources distributed. In the more collective society characteristic of the twentieth century much of society's energies were invested in just such argument and debate. A major part of personal identity was whether one stood on the left or right of the political divide, and whether society should be socialist or capitalist. Public life was shaped by the major political parties around the 'big questions' of who should own what, and why. Connected to the fragmentation of wider ties and associations, politics has lost much of its meaning and instead tends to latch on to, and express individual insecurities.[48] Government policy initiatives such as NHS helplines instinctively seek to reconnect with the public through the only aspirations that one can take for granted in a non-political society: personal health and survival. Official endorsement for these preoccupations endows them with authority and credibility beyond the individual.

Intermediate, contextual factors

Lack of contexual knowledge

To an extent, the characteristics of risk objects do have a bearing on the possibility of alarm being generated, but this is likely to be because of a contextual lack of knowledge rather than because it is known what is threatening. The continued mystery of autism is central to understanding the impact made by the false link with the childhood vaccine, MMR, for example. It is partially because science currently still knows so little about autism that it is possible for unfounded theories to make such an impact – particularly among parents desperate to understand their children's condition. Lack of scientific understanding in other cases such as BSE provides the opportunity for alarmist ideas to develop.

Temporal coincidence with other alarming issues

When more than one worrying development follows another, there is the potential for a greater sense of a threat and loss of perspective. Take the example of the SARS virus. Its actual impact was relatively modest and localised, not least because it could not be transmitted so easily as flu. In historical terms this virulent new virus was most striking for the speed with which it was identified and isolated in the period from March to June 2003. Yet, notwithstanding limited media shaping of frames of reference, the virus generated panic in some societies, at considerable economic cost.[49] An important factor that explains the disproportionate reaction was that it happened in the climate of fear generated by 9/11 and the 'war on terror' mindset that followed. There is the potential for a 'scenario' being created when alarms coincide, as opposed to single, manageable issues.

Legacy issues

The potential for alarm is strongly influenced by so called legacy issues: the cumulative impact of previous, connected concerns in the past. Although it is a misleading label, mobile phones use a (harmless, 'non-ionising') form of 'radiation' and this worrying connection is an important factor in framing how the issue is understood. Similarly, anything related to the stigmatised terms 'genetic' and 'chemicals' are similarly liable, unless the association is consciously broken.

Actors' role in constructing alarm and trigger moments

'Risk entrepreneurs'

The risk society has encouraged the emergence of 'actors' dedicated to the promotion of particular risks. Particular individuals and institutions have enhanced their profile and prestige through identification with particular concerns and it is in their interest to maintain their issue's profile. For example, Dr Andrew Wakefield almost single-handedly instigated the alarm over MMR. The lead quotations from stories identifying mobile phones with health problems in the British media came from three individuals. While they do not necessarily stand to gain financially, the identities and sense of purpose of 'risk entrepreneurs' become bound up with a continued high profile for their chosen concern.

Campaigners

The role of campaign groups in the promotion of particular risk anxieties has been recognised, if unexplored, since Douglas and Wildavsky's *Risk and Culture*.[50] Consumer and environmental groups were central to the emergence of a risk-averse culture in the USA. They remain central to many contemporary risk alarms, such as over GM foods and the corresponding promotion of risk avoidance through more regulation. Given their sometimes high profile, their role can be exaggerated, however. Without the preconditions and some of the intermediate variables above, and flattery by more important, state actors it is unlikely that their actions could be influential.

The media

The media have been central not only to the dissemination of risk alarms, but sometimes their virtual creation. This is hardly surprising given that concerns such as those over radiation from mobile phones have no basis in everyday knowledge or experience, and can only be brought in from without. In the UK, in particular, the media have been central to many key risk alarms. An edition of the television show, *Watchdog*, in November 1988 concerned the theory that eggs were responsible for increases in food poisoning and created the pressure that led to alarm. An edition of the same programme was similarly central to the mobile phone alarm. However, the role of the media varies greatly from issue to issue, and is sometimes liable to be exaggerated. In the case of SARS the media played a more incidental role, whilst in the MMR alarm an active role in undermining risk – it was through the investigations of journalist Brian Deer for the *Sunday Times* newspaper that Andrew Wakefield was exposed and fatally undermined.[51]

Official responses

The least widely examined, but arguably most important response that shapes subsequent reactions is that of official authority and expertise. This is unsurprising as even in a cynical and mistrustful age we expect the relevant authorities to take primary responsibility for any potential crisis. By comparison, no matter how alarmist the calls of risk entrepreneurs, campaign groups and the media, their role is unlikely to be decisive in itself, independently of how the authorities respond. The decisive role of authority can be seen in the number of alarms that have been specifically instigated by official statements and policy approaches. In December 1988, for example, the then Junior Health Minister, Edwina Currie, uttered 20 words in a television interview, sparking a food scare crisis that temporarily crippled an industry: 'We do warn people now that most of the egg production in this country, sadly, is now infected with salmonella'.[52] The fact that her words, in themselves, were mild and hardly alarmist underlines the centrality of official risk communication.

Trigger moments and premature scientific revelation

Finally it is important to recognise the impact made by a particular (preventable) moment in the creation of risk alarms. Edwina Currie's statement is a classic example; had this statement not been made it is unlikely a crisis over salmonella would have ensued. Further, it is possible to identify a common pattern to many of the most important contemporary risk alarms that was set by the early example of salmonella. A common characteristic of such trigger moments is the sudden revelation of a dramatic theory about a potential risk that has not been subject to considered scientific scrutiny and debate. When Andrew Wakefield held the press conference at which the theory of MMR's link to autism was announced, an alarm was made. In less dramatic fashion, the alarm over the human form of 'mad cow disease' was triggered by the public revelation of the possible link at a time when it could have little possible consequence other than alarm.

With hindsight these new theories have turned out to be of varying value. What can be said is that some were announced without clear regard for the possible consequences, or for the established process of other scientists checking new ideas. Risk alarms are ultimately born of a nervousness and uncertainty among authorities about how they should now manage anything that might be perceived as a threat to public health. Increasingly, the sensible course of action from the perspective of those in scientific and political authority has been one of shifting potential blame and responsibility elsewhere by immediately placing even uncertain knowledge into the public domain. In the environment of the 'risk society' this has often resulted in alarm and further uncertainty.

Conclusion

Health risk alarms are not isolated incidents but form part of an important pattern in modern societies. They have only arisen during the last 40 years, first of all in the USA. They need to be understood in the wider context of a 'risk society' marked by greater choice and individualisation but weaker trust and belief in progress. The relative strength of such characteristics influences the propensity for risk alarms. Understanding why Americans are happy to grow and eat genetically modified crops while Britons are more cautious, for example, is partially explained by the more pro-scientific outlook and greater optimism about the future that prevails in the USA. The stronger social solidarity still found within many European countries tends to counter the tendency to alarms about paedophiles within the community. Such alarms are not only a product of these forces, but actively reinforce a culture of mistrust and the erosion of informality. Awareness of risks is not simply common sense avoidance of clear dangers. It is also a demonstration of being a responsible citizen in a post-political society where staying healthy has become an end in itself.

Risks cannot be understood in their own terms. It is the social, political and cultural context that determines what is perceived as a risk, and whether an alarm is triggered. Risk alarms are not only the product of wider social trends and forces, but are actively made by particular individuals and institutions. Most decisive is the approach taken by relevant state and government bodies; although they may perceive their actions as a response to events, they are in fact the key to how society responds. The generally very defensive reaction of state authority to risk concerns in the late modern period has created a risk-averse society that sometimes appears afraid even of its own shadow.

Discussion topics

- Why has the avoidance of health risks become a moral imperative in British society?
- Does it matter if society is becoming more averse to risk?
- How might the rising trend in risk alarms be reversed?

Further reading

Burgess, A. (2004) *Cellular Phones, Public Fears and a Culture of Precaution*. Cambridge: Cambridge University Press.

This is a contemporary case study in the creation of a risk alarm that is very accessible and provides interesting historical and national comparisons on a familiar issue.

Douglas, M. and Wildavsky, A. (1982) *Risk and Culture*. London: University of California Press.

This remains the most thought-provoking reflection on risk alarms, also providing a crucial reminder of how they first emerged in the USA.

Furedi, F. (1997) *The Culture of Fear*. London: Cassell.

This study dramatically outlines the social processes involved and the social consequences of a society bounded by risk.

Giddens, A. *The Runaway World: Risk*. BBC Reith Lectures. Available at: http://news.bbc.co.uk/hi/english/static/events/reith_99/week2/week2.htm.

This short lecture by Anthony Giddens is useful in historically locating risk and summaring key issues.

References

1 Douglas, M. and Wildavsky, A. (1982) *Risk and Culture*. London: University of California Press.
2 Burgess, A. (2004) *Cellular Phones, Public Fears and a Culture of Precaution*. Cambridge: Cambridge University Press, p. 99.
3 Porritt, J. (2000) *Playing Safe: Science and the Environment*. London: Thames and Hudson.
4 Beck, U. (1992) *Risk Society: Towards a New Modernity*. London: Sage.
5 Burgess, A. (2006) The making of the risk-centred society and the limits of social risk research. *Health, Risk and Society*, 8(4): 329–42.
6 Fitzpatrick, M. (2004) *MMR and Autism: What Every Parent Needs to Know*. London: Routledge.
7 Alcock, R. and Busby, J. (2006) Risk migration and scientific advance: the case of flame-retardant compounds. *Risk Analysis*, 26(2): 369–81.
8 Quigley, K. (2005) Bug reactions: Considering US government and UK government Y2K operations in light of media coverage and public opinion polls. *Health, Risk & Society*, 7(3): 267–91.
9 Hargreaves, I., Lewis, J. and Speers, T. (2003) *Towards a Better Map: Science, the Public and the Media*. Swindon: ESRC.
10 Reilly, J. (1999) Just another food scare? Public understanding and the BSE crisis. In Greg Philo (ed.), *Message Received*. New York: Longman, p. 129.
11 See Special Issue: Media, Crisis and SARS of the *Asian Journal of Communication*, 15(3).
12 Burgess, A. (2004) ibid.
13 Slovic, P. (1987) Perception of risk. *Science*, 230: 280–5.
14 Independent Expert Group on Mobile Phones (2000) *Mobile Phones and Health*. Didcot: NRPB. Available at: http://www.iegmp.org.uk/
15 Burgess, A. (2006) ibid.
16 Emsley, J. (1994) *The Consumer's Good Chemical Guide*. Oxford: W.H. Freeman.
17 Campos, P. (2004) *The Obesity Myth*. New York: Gotham Books.
18 Ericson, R. and Doyle, A. (2003) *Risk and Morality*. Toronto: University of Toronto Press.

19 Douglas, M. and Wildavsky, A. (1982) ibid.
20 Dogan, M. (1998) The decline of traditional values in Western Europe. *International Journal of Comparative Sociology,* 39(1): 77–90.
21 RSA Commission on Illegal Drugs (2007) *Drugs: Facing Facts.* London: RSA. Available at: http://www.rsadrugscommission.org/
22 Jenkins, N. (2006) 'You can't wrap them up in cotton wool!' Constructing risk in young people's access to outdoor play. *Health, Risk & Society,* 8(4): 379–93.
23 Pain, R. et al. (2005) So long as I take my mobile phone: mobile phones, urban life and geographies of young people's safety. *International Journal of Urban and Regional Research,* 29(4): 814–30.
24 Fukuyama, F. (1995) *Trust.* London: Penguin.
25 Jenkins, P. (1999) *Synthetic Panics: The Symbolic Politics of Designer Drugs.* New York: New York University Press.
26 Furedi, F. (1997) *The Culture of Fear.* London: Cassell.
27 Piper, H., Powell, J. and Smith, H. (2006) Parents, professionals and paranoia: the touching of children in a culture of fear. *Journal of Social Work,* 6(2): 151–67.
28 Giddens, A. (1999) *The Runaway World: Risk.* BBC Reith Lectures. Available at: http://news.bbc.co.uk/hi/english/static/events/reith_99/week2/week2.htm
29 Green, J. (1997) *Risk and Misfortune: The Social Construction of Accidents.* London: University of California Press.
30 Thomas, K. (1997) Health and morality in early modern England. In A. Brandt and P. Rozin (eds), *Morality and Health.* London: Routledge.
31 Bernstein, P. (1998) *Against the Gods: The Remarkable Story of Risk.* London: John Wiley.
32 Furedi, F. (1997) ibid.
33 Porritt, J. (2000) ibid.
34 Starr, C. (1969) Social benefit versus technological risk. *Science,* 165: 1232.
35 Slovic, P. (1987) ibid.
36 Townsend, E. and Campbell, S. (2004) Psychological determinants of willingness to taste and purchase GM food. *Risk Analysis,* 24(5): 1385–93.
37 Frewer, L.J., Miles, S. and Marsh, R. (2002) The media and genetically modified foods: evidence in support of social amplification of risk. *Risk Analysis,* 22(4): 701–11.
38 Hargreaves, I., Lewis, J. and Speers, T. (2003) *Towards a Better Map: Science, the Public and the Media.* Swindon: ESRC.
39 diFonzo, N. and Prashant, B. (2002) Corporate rumour activity, belief and practice. *Public Relations Review,* 28: 1–19.
40 Barnett, J. et al. (in press) Public responses to precautionary information from the Department of Health about possible health risks from mobile phones. *Health Policy.*
41 Beck, U. (1992) *Risk Society: Towards a New Modernity.* London: Sage.
42 Giddens, A. ibid.
43 Pidgeon, N., Kasperson, R. and Slovic, P. (2003) *The Social Amplification of Risk.* Cambridge: Cambridge University Press.
44 Inglehart, R. (1971) The silent revolution in post-industrial societies. *American Political Science Review,* 65: 991–1017, or Inglehart, R. (1977) *The Silent Revolution: Changing Values and Political Styles Among Western Publics.* Princeton, NJ: Princeton University Press.
45 Durodie, B. (2003) The true cost of precautionary chemicals regulation. *Risk Analysis,* 23(2): 389–98.

46 Bellah, R. et al. (1985) *Habits of the Heart: Individualism and Commitment in American Life*. Berkeley, CA: University of California Press.

47 Jacoby, R. (1999) *The End of Utopia*. New York: Basic Books.

48 Boggs, C. (2001) *The End of Politics*. New York: Guildford Press.

49 Smith, R. (2005) *Infectious Disease and Risk: Lessons from SARS*. London: Nuffield Trust Global Programme on Health, Foreign Policy and Security.

50 Douglas, M. and Wildavsky, A. (1982) ibid.

51 Fitzpatrick, M. (2004) ibid.

52 North, R. and Gorman, T. (1990) *Chickengate: An Independent Investigation of the Salmonella in Eggs Scare*. London: IEA.

5

Illness Behaviour and the Discourse of Health

David Wainwright

- Sociologist's distinguish between *disease* – the presence of physical pathology, and *illness* – the patient's subjective experience of symptoms.
- *Illness behaviour* – includes all of the disturbances to an individual's life which stem from the experience of illness, including changes in functioning and activity, and uptake of health services and other welfare benefits.
- The *discourse of health* refers to the totality of cultural norms, expectations and technologies through which a society understands and responds to illness.
- Changes in the discourse of health have given rise to forms of illness behaviour for which little evidence of physical pathology can be found.
- This epidemic of *medically unexplained symptoms* has been accompanied by the development of new strategies for governing health and illness.

> If I'd known I was going to live this long I'd have taken better care of myself.
> Jazz pianist Eubie Blake shortly before his 100th birthday

Mrs Lancaster's injury

On 5 July 1999 Beverley Lancaster left Birmingham County Court with £67,000 in compensation for a 'stress-related personal injury'. Mrs Lancaster had worked as a draughtsman at Birmingham City Council, but when her post was abolished she was redeployed as a part-time housing officer. As a draughtsman Mrs Lancaster had not dealt with the public, but her new role entailed dealing with council tenants who could be abusive. The Council had promised training, but despite several requests this was not provided.

Within three months Mrs Lancaster found that she could not cope and took two lengthy periods of sick leave, eventually retiring on grounds of ill health. Commenting on the case, the head of legal services at Mrs Lancaster's trade union claimed that:

> Initially it was quite difficult to bring the case to court because people are quite dismissive of stress at work. But now employers know that if they damage the

minds of their employees, they will have to pay out in the same way as if they did not repair the stairs and someone fell down and broke a leg.[1]

Following the trial Mrs Lancaster returned to work as a school assistant for children with special needs, although she felt that the stress she endured had done her lasting harm. 'The pay-out is great,' she said, 'but it can't compensate for what I've had to face up to: the fact that going to work made me ill.'[2]

Mrs Lancaster's injury raises questions about health and illness at the turn of the millennium. Why are problems of everyday life, such as coping with the demands of a new job, experienced as health problems? The trade union officer claimed that emotional distress is equivalent to a broken leg, but is injury or illness fundamentally a description of physical changes in the body, or is it a way of behaving in the world which can exist independently of organic pathology? If illness resides in behaviour rather than organic disease then who is responsible for its occurrence: the person exhibiting it or the external agents or circumstances that provoked it?

These questions apply not just to Mrs Lancaster's injury, nor just to her fellow work stress sufferers, but to a large and growing group of people who suffer from new illnesses many of which would have been unrecognisable to their grandparents. The issues they raise are central to the contemporary experience of health and illness in the developed world. The aim of this chapter is to explain the emergence of these new forms of illness at this specific point in time. Our analysis begins with what is perhaps the keystone of medical sociology – the claim that disease and illness are two things rather than one.

Disease and illness

The bio-medical model of *disease* emerged from the Enlightenment belief in the application of science to the solution of human problems, but the medical model is not a fixed set of beliefs suspended in amber since the nineteenth century, indeed its defining characteristic is the constancy of change as better knowledge of physiology is revealed.[3] Nor is medical practice confined to the bio-medical model; doctors use a range of interpretations and practices which lie outside of clinical science, and their assumptions about the nature of illness and disease have broadened to include insights gleaned from other disciplines. Even so, both supporters and critics of the medical model would recognise it as an ideal type and agree on its primacy in western healthcare.

The medical model is *materialist*, and assumes that the mechanisms of the body can be revealed and understood in the same way that the workings of the solar system can be understood through gazing at the night sky; by theories derived from rigorous observation. The grounding of medical knowledge in empirical observation, rather than philosophical abstraction, differentiates modern medicine from its predecessors. The ability to look inside the body has enabled modern medicine to classify and understand diseases by observing pathogenic agents at work, for instance, with infectious diseases, bacterial or viral organisms can be observed attacking the cells of the body. This physiological pathway can be traced to observable physical symptoms, for example, the actions of the common cold virus on the cells of the body can be traced through to the onset of coughing and sneezing.

The scientific methods employed in the compilation of medical knowledge are not foolproof, even dissection can produce knowledge which is invalid. During the nineteenth century the corpses of poverty-stricken inmates of London's workhouses were used to teach anatomy in the city's medical schools. Today it is recognised that extreme poverty often enlarges the adrenal glands, but during the nineteenth century these pathological changes were mistakenly classified as normal. On the rare occasions when corpses of the rich were dissected they were found to have 'abnormally' small adrenal glands and a new disease classification – idiopathic adrenal atrophy – was invented to label this apparent disease.[4] Scientific knowledge may also be distorted by prevailing cultural assumptions, for example, the disease of 'drapetomania' was constructed to explain why slaves often ran away from their owners,[5] and medical knowledge has often been implicated in the social control of women.[6] However, such errors are rare and it is through more rigorous observation and application of the scientific method that they are recognised and corrected.

As well as generating a system of disease classification based on rigorous observation, the bio-medical model also provides a systematic strategy for diagnosing and treating disease, sometimes explained through the metaphor of a 'faulty machine'. A fault is identified or diagnosed by observing symptoms or conducting diagnostic tests, a theory of what caused the fault is developed, an intervention is prescribed to repair the fault, and the outcome is measured to test the adequacy of the diagnostic theory. The bio-medical model is not just a formulaic body of knowledge, but a scientific method of clinical practice which uses observation, generation of hypotheses and empirical testing.[7]

Bio-medical science lies behind modern medicine's spectacular advances in the war against disease, but is disease the *only* factor that explains how people behave when they are ill?

Medical sociologists draw a distinction between *disease*, defined as the presence of a physical abnormality, and *illness*, defined as the experience of symptoms, the meanings ascribed to them, and associated forms of behaviour including help seeking and changes in role performance.[8,9] The bio-medical model assumes that *illness behaviour* is a direct response to physical pathology; the individual contracts a disease or injury which causes them to respond and behave in a given way, for example a broken leg will necessarily entail pain, impaired ability to walk and some form of clinical intervention in order to heal successfully. While physical pathology can be a powerful determinant of illness behaviour social factors are also important. This conclusion was arrived at through empirical observation of *social variations* in illness behaviour.

In the early 1950s, Zborowski found variations in the response to pain exhibited by different ethnic groups attending New York City Hospital.[10] Where 'Old Americans' tended to respond with stoicism and Irish patients denied their pain, Italian subjects were more concerned about obtaining pain relief, and Jewish patients with what the pain meant and its significance for their future health. Zborowski explained these differences in terms of the ways that different ethnic groups socialised their children:

The child learns to pay attention to each painful experience and to look for help and sympathy which are readily given to him. In Jewish families, where not only a slight sensation of pain but also each deviation from the child's normal behaviour is looked upon as a sign of illness, the child is prone to acquire anxieties with regard to the meaning and significance of these manifestations.[11]

The response to physical symptoms is not a direct function of disease or injury; it is also influenced by the ways in which people make sense of their symptoms and choose to act. This process of 'making sense' is not exclusively conditioned by individual traits, but is the product of shared cultural beliefs and expectations exchanged within the individual's social network. Decisions about when to seek medical advice are influenced by advice from family and friends or the 'lay referral' system.[12]

Illness behaviour also varies between classes. Koos found that middle-class people were more likely to exhibit illness and help-seeking behaviour than working-class people with the same symptoms.[13] Decisions about whether to become ill or seek medical advice are often weighed against competing demands from family and work and the financial consequences of becoming ill.[14,15] In their study of working-class mothers Blaxter and Paterson found that children's symptoms were only recognised as illness if they impaired the child's ability to walk or play, with functionally insignificant symptoms dismissed as normal.[16]

Since the 1950s, social variations in illness behaviour have been extensively documented, however, the mechanism by which these factors exert their influence is poorly understood.[17] The difficulty in arriving at a comprehensive theory of illness behaviour stems from a fundamental problem in social philosophy which relates to the dichotomy of 'free-will and determinism', or 'structure and agency'.[18] Sociologists reject biological reductionism, and recognise that social factors are also important, but if people behave differently in response to objectively similar symptoms, does this imply that such behaviour is freely chosen, or is it simply a response to a different set of determinants, that is social factors rather than physiological ones? Variations in illness behaviour imply that ethnic group, social class and gender are powerful determinants, but this observation can lead to the adoption of a social determinist model of illness behaviour that is as mechanistic as the biological reductionism of the medical model.

What biological and social determinist models both fail to recognise is the extent to which illness behaviour is mediated by consciousness. There may be strong physiological factors pushing someone towards illness behaviour, and equally strong social factors channelling the form that illness behaviour will take, but within the constraints imposed by even the severest forms of physical pathology and the most adverse social circumstances, humans still possess the capacity to choose how to act.[19]

The social philosopher Margaret Archer[20] refers to this as 'the internal conversation' and it applies well to the decision making that underpins illness behaviour, for example, the individual who wakes with a hangover is confronted by a series of choices: whether to stay in bed, or get up and go to work, whether to self-medicate, or seek professional help. These choices might be constrained by the severity of the symptoms, or by consideration of the social and economic consequences of becoming ill: "Will I lose money if I don't go to work?', 'Who will take the children to school if I stay in bed?', 'What will my family and friends think of me if I succumb to illness?'. This internal conversation may also be influenced by group norms or broader cultural beliefs: "Is it normal for someone like me to take a day off work?', 'Am I the type of person who stays in bed with a hangover?' This internal conversation is not easily resolved, nor are the actions which stem from it easily accomplished. The physical reality of the impaired body can frustrate our most deeply held plans and the force of social factors can also undermine our projects. Negotiating the physical and social imperatives towards health or illness can be a struggle, but it is the human capacity to engage in this struggle that lies behind notions of *resilience* and courage.

That illness is not simply a direct function of disease, but the result of a complex web of physical, social, and cultural factors, is perhaps the most significant claim of medical sociology. Chapter 1 examined how these insights have given rise to different social models of health, including: the *'social determinants of health'* perspective; the *'unhealthy lifestyles'* approach; and the different strands of *'social consructionism'*. Since the mid-twentieth century social models of health and illness have grown in influence; resonating beyond the academic realm to influence the popular discourse of health. Not only has this changed health policy and medical practice, it has also changed popular definitions of illness and given rise to new forms of illness behaviour. The following section explores the ways in which the discourse of health has been transformed by the incorporation of social models of illness.

The changing discourse of health

The discourse of health refers to the totality of cultural norms, expectations and technologies through which a society understands and responds to illness. An obvious criticism is that this implies a consensus that cannot be found in reality, for instance, a general practitioner may have an understanding of the social influences on health which is different to that of a neurologist, and the pronouncements of the Royal Colleges may have little resonance for doctors lower in the professional hierarchy.[21] Include not just other health professions, politicians, and policy makers, but also the broader population, and the notion of a *single* discourse of health becomes difficult to sustain.

The discourse of health cannot refer to a fixed set of beliefs and practices uniformly subscribed to by all, but must encompass differences and contradictions, varying not just between individuals, groups and places, but also over time. Mapping these differences is a valuable exercise, but focusing on the *micro*-sociology of health beliefs may overlook broader processes of change that occur at the *macro* level – a case of not seeing the wood for the trees. Take for example, Mrs Lancaster's problem of work stress; there is within the discourse of health considerable disagreement over the nature of work stress, its causes and how it should be dealt with, but the category of work stress is recognisable and available for contestation in contemporary western societies in a way which it was not in, say, the 1930s.[22] Only by moving from the micro level of personal problems to the macro level of social issues can the sociological imagination reflect on these broad transformations and their implications for everyday life.[23] This is the analytical justification for persevering with the notion of the discourse of health – although the category necessarily lacks specificity and precision, it is essential to the project of recognising and understanding broad patterns of social change.

The social models have permeated the discourse of health via several routes, but two areas are particularly important in terms of the inflation of illness behaviour: first is the emergence of the *New Public Health* movement, and the second is the adoption of *Patient-centred Practice* which has altered the doctor–patient relationship, particularly in general practice where over 90 per cent of patient contacts occur.

The New Public Health

For at least a century public health has provided the vehicle through which social models of health have influenced health policy. As curative medicine expanded during the twentieth century with increased spending on hospitals and high-technology medicine, the public health lobby argued for an alternative strategy of population-based disease prevention and health promotion.

Although spending on public health policies remains small in comparison with acute services, it has had a substantial influence on shared beliefs about the meaning of health. A key moment came in 1946 when the World Health Organisation (WHO) redefined health as 'a state of complete physical, mental and social well-being, and not merely the absence of disease or infirmity'.[24] A clear indictment of the bio-medical model with its emphasis on organic disease, its neglect of the subjective experiences of the patient and the role of social influences on health. However, the WHO's redefinition coincided with the beginning of a golden age of clinical science[25] and it was another 30 years before the *New Public Health* (NPH) emerged as a serious challenge to the dominance of bio-medical orthodoxy.

In 1977 the WHO and UNICEF launched a campaign demanding *Health For All by the Year 2000* (HFA 2000) at a conference in Alma Ata. The declaration provided a rallying point for a new generation of health and welfare professionals, radicalised in the late 1960s and early 1970s, who were growing disillusioned with the exhaustion of traditional strategies for social change.[26] The NPH proposed that social justice could be pursued through professional activities such as health needs assessment and community empowerment.[27]

This political division was underlined by publication of the Report of a Research Working Party into Inequalities of Health, chaired by Douglas Black and subsequently referred to as the Black Report.[28] Commissioned by a Labour Government in 1977, but reporting to the newly elected Conservative administration in 1980, the report charted the widening gap in mortality rates between the richest and poorest social classes, and proposed a substantial extension of the welfare state to close the gap. It is difficult to find a working party whose findings were more at odds with the ideology of the government to which it reported. In a foreword penned by the Secretary of State for Social Services, Patrick Jenkins, the recommendations were dismissed as too expensive, and adding a whiff of suppression, the report was issued on a Bank Holiday in the form of 250 photocopies.

Though the Black Report's recommendations were not implemented, its findings coupled with the hostile response from government catalysed the NPH, stimulating a wave of further research. At a time when old political strategies were crumbling, the aim of reducing health inequalities offered a clearly defined project which could be pursued, not as a political campaign, but as a neutral programme of scientific enquiry and professional practice. Throughout the 1980s and early 1990s advocates of the NPH were active in governmental and quasi-governmental agencies at the international, national and local levels, and WHO continued its HFA 2000 campaign, with the setting of national targets for European countries in 1985. During this period the relationship between the NPH and government changed from one of antagonism to one of increasing collaboration. This rapprochement entailed adjustment on both sides. For the NPH programme to be acceptable to government it had to be purged of its commitment to radical structural change and expansion of the old-style welfare state, but by the same token in order to embrace the NPH agenda, the Conservative government had to dilute its opposition to state intervention in the personal lives of its citizens. This process of mutual adjustment quickened in the early 1980s with the emergence of a decidedly old-fashioned threat to public health in the form of HIV/AIDS.

Where the Black Report's emphasis on inequality was anathema to the Conservatives, the government had fewer objections to launching a campaign against the dangers of sexual promiscuity. In 1987 the *Don't Die of Ignorance* initiative was launched. As well as national advertising, resources were invested in 'HIV co-ordinators' and other health promotion professionals, whose responsibilities initially included the promotion of 'safe sex' among 'high-risk groups' such as gay men and intravenous drug users, transforming over time to the promotion of 'safer sex' among 'at risk' groups – virtually anyone who was sexually active outside of a stable monogamous relationship.

The AIDS campaign had two important consequences for the changing discourse of health. First, it contributed to a heightened sense of personal vulnerability. Government epidemiologists produced inflated estimates of the anticipated epidemic, claiming that within a decade everyone would know someone who had died from the disease.[29] Second, the AIDS campaign corroded the boundary between public and personal life. The Conservative government may not have objected to the pathologisation of extra-marital sex, but the AIDS campaign went much further than traditional forms of moral regulation, breaking long-established taboos about public discussion of sexual activity, and opening the private relationship between sexual partners to governance by the state.[30] This cycle of identifying a potential health risk, amplifying public perceptions of vulnerability, and developing policy initiatives to regulate the risk, has been constantly repeated since the mid-1980s in health scares about: 'mad cow disease'; sunbathing and skin cancer; the dangers of mobile phone use; as well as traditional health promotion topics of diet, smoking and alcohol.

By the late 1980s the reorientation of the NPH away from demands for structural change, towards the politically neutral field of health promotion was well underway. By 1988 the Chief Medical Officer Donald Acheson was able to recommend an extended role for Public Health doctors and endorse the WHO's approach of setting targets for public health.[31] Following the demise of Mrs Thatcher, the assimilation of the NPH into government policy took another step forward, when her successor John Major and his Minister for Health, Virginia Bottomley, announced the *Health of the Nation* strategy (Green Paper 1991, White Paper 1992).

Health of the Nation was cautiously welcomed by radical advocates of the NPH as an important first step towards embracing the WHO's *HFA 2000* agenda. Even health inequalities were no longer taboo, although referred to by the less contentious label of *variations in health*. However, rather than ushering in a new age of radicalism *Health of the Nation* marked the final separation of the NPH from its radical roots. The Black Report's recommendations for wealth redistribution and increased welfare benefits were ignored in favour of individualised health promotion campaigns often mediated by community groups.

Health of the Nation represented the effective co-option of the NPH into government policy; shorn of its radical origins and equipped with a new operational arm of intermediary agencies that occupied a space between the formal institutions of the state and the informal groupings of civil society. This new apparatus for the regulation of everyday life may have been largely in place by the mid-1990s, but residual suspicions about the 'nanny state' and 'coercive healthism'[32] continued to restrain Conservative Health Ministers from making full use of it. In 1997 a New Labour government was elected that had no such reservations.

Apart from appointing a Minister for Public Health, the Labour government's early public health policy continued in much the same vein as that of the previous administration. A White Paper in 1999, *Saving Lives*,[33] introduced *Health Action Zones* and a more extensive smoking cessation programme, effectively extending the apparatus developed by the Conservatives. However, although *Saving Lives* originated in the Department of Health it was signed by nine other ministers, indicating the need for 'joined up government' to tackle the problems of public health. The notion that health is an outcome of broad social and economic factors is central to NPH discourse and its proponents would not have a problem with other government ministries joining the drive towards health improvement. However, the intra-governmental collaboration expanded beyond pursuit of the health targets revised in *Saving Lives*, it marked the expansion of the individualised therapeutic model of health promotion into virtually all aspects of social policy.

Emblematic of this expansion was the *Social Exclusion Unit* set up in 1997 to coordinate the new government's policies on poverty. As Fitzpatrick has argued, adoption of the term social exclusion in preference to poverty, marks more than just a change in language.[34] 'Poverty' is grounded in material disadvantage and evokes the social democratic agenda of wealth redistribution and welfarism. Social exclusion is concerned with how inequality is subjectively experienced by the individual, with its effects on self-esteem and the behaviour of those affected. This transition has its origins in the health inequalities debate, where social stressors are seen as potent sources of emotional and physical strain, and unhealthy lifestyle choices. The evolution of the NPH entailed a shift from redistributive solutions to poverty, towards interventions aimed at managing emotional states and individual behaviour. Under New Labour this therapeutic approach to health policy has been applied to a much wider range of social problems, including: reduction of teenage pregnancies, improvement of educational attainment, and the control of anti-social behaviour.

Furedi refers to this process as the development of a 'therapy culture' in which health and social problems are increasingly explained in terms of the individual's inability to satisfactorily govern his own emotional and mental life, for example, 'low self-esteem' has become a potent folk myth invoked to explain virtually all social problems.[35] Furedi notes that in the USA there has been a backlash against self-esteem interventions, with several studies suggesting that unconditional flattery and unwarranted praise have created a generation of self-centred 'brats' whose performance at school and subsequent behaviour has deteriorated. Whether raising self-esteem is seen as a solution or a problem, both arguments assume that the basis of social and health problems resides in the individual's inability to adequately manage their emotional and mental life. This orientation effectively locates much of social policy within the broadened discourse of health.

The NPH has come a long way from its radical roots. The demands for social change and extension of the welfare state have largely been abandoned in order to obtain greater influence over government policy. An orientation towards the social determinants of health has been retained, but the focus has shifted towards the identification of 'risk factors', giving rise to a heightened sense of vulnerability and the extension of therapeutic intervention into new areas of everyday life. The effect of the NPH on the discourse of health has been profound; however, other developments have also had a significant impact. We turn now to the adoption of the patient-centered approach to general practice.

Patient-centred practice

The rapid increase in the efficacy of hospital-based medicine in the post-war period provoked a crisis within general practice. By the early 1960s generalists were widely viewed as the 'poor relations' of hospital consultants, largely left behind by the revolution in high-technology medicine and lacking the status and rewards of their colleagues in the acute sector.[36] This crisis coincided with the emergence of social models of health which provided useful material from which general practice could reinvent itself. Critics had long argued that bio-medicine should be complemented by a holistic approach which addressed the patient's subjective experiences and social circumstances.[37,38] The Peckham Health Centre experiment of the 1930s had complemented traditional medical services with cultural and exercise facilities,[39] but failed to take root and it was not until the rise of the New Public Health that general practice became re-engaged with health promotion. Since the *Health of the Nation* strategy was introduced in 1992, successive governments have extended the responsibilities of general practitioners for health promotion and preventive medicine, despite the ambivalence of the profession.[40] However, the impact of social models of health on general practice is more profound than government's attempts to embroil GPs in health promotion.

From the late 1960s general practitioners began to redefine their discipline in terms of holism and the psycho-social model. Michael Balint's *The Doctor, His Patient and the Illness*,[41] was particularly influential, arguing that effective general practice depended upon a rich understanding of the patient's social circumstances and the ways in which he made sense of life events and experiences. Rather than focusing exclusively on physiology the doctor must engage with the patient as a conscious thinking subject; in effect adopting a patient-centred approach.

The rationale for patient-centred practice stems from the limitations of the traditional medical model in addressing the full gamut of human suffering. Biological reductionism might underpin the greatest achievements of modern medicine in combating disease, but it has proven less effective in tackling the subjective aspects of illness, and it is argued that in order to fully address the psycho-social aspects of human suffering medical practice must forsake traditional mind–body dualism.[42] For instance, Smith argues that successful pain management depends on not just the dispensing of analgesia but also on medical practitioners making socio-economic factors and psychosomatic experiences a part of their clinical concern.[43] The medical anthropologist Arthur Kleinman has attempted to integrate this approach into clinical practice by conducting 'mini ethnographies' of patients which it is claimed leads to more humane care through 'the empathic witnessing of [their] existential experiences of suffering and practical coping with the psycho-social crises that constitute the menacing chronicity of that experience'.[44]

The belief that healing is an art as well as a science has a long history in western medicine, particularly in relation to the role of the family doctor; however, post-Balint general practice is characterised by a radical recasting of the doctor–patient relationship which has undermined the general practitioner's authority to police the boundary between illness and health and act as an effective gatekeeper to the uptake of health services and other health-related welfare benefits.

When the patient was conceptualised as a set of physiological signs and symptoms to be diagnosed and treated by the doctor using the expert knowledge and skills conferred by clinical science, the views of the patient were likely to be seen by both parties as secondary to those of the doctor. The adoption of a patient-centred approach turns this traditional relationship on its head. No longer a passive object subordinated to clinical authority, the patient's experiences and interpretations become the key to defining the illness and selecting an appropriate treatment. In the 1970s medical sociologists explored the problem of *patient compliance* with the course of treatment prescribed by the doctor.[45] Today emphasis has shifted from the paternalistic notion of compliance, to the more egalitarian principle of *concordance*, in which doctor and patient share their 'knowledge' of the problem and agree a mutually acceptable course of action.[46] The recent 'expert patient' initiative takes this redistribution of power one step further, suggesting that the chronically ill may understand their illness better than their doctor.[47]

The elevation of subjective experiences of illness over objective evidence of pathology has introduced a dilemma into diagnosis. What to do if no evidence of pathology can be found, yet the patient persists in viewing the illness as essentially organic rather than psycho-social in origin?[48] The dilemma is all the more vexed because many patients appear to conflate a psycho-social diagnosis with a diminution of the seriousness of their complaint or even as a moral judgement on their lack of resilience. This is the great irony of the patient-centred approach: by definition it confers a great deal of explanatory power on patients' subjective beliefs and interpretations, yet when patients are empowered in this way they often deny the possibility of a psycho-social explanation of their illness and insist that they are suffering from organic disease. Having adopted a patient-centred approach the doctor cannot revert to clinical science to debunk the patient's illness claim without running the risk of invalidating the patient, thereby potentially adding to the patient's suffering and damaging the doctor–patient relationship.

This diminished capacity to reject illness claims which cannot be explained by reference to observable pathology has substantially inflated illness behaviour. Kroenke and Mangelsdorff's retrospective review of case notes in a US ambulatory care clinic (broadly equivalent to British general practice) found that the 14 symptoms most commonly reported to generalists could only be medically explained in a minority of cases, for example, chest pain, headache, back pain and abdominal pain could only be medically explained in 10 per cent of cases.[49] Hamilton et al. applied a similar methodology to outpatient clinics in the UK and found the following rates of medically unexplained cases: gastroenterology 53 per cent, neurology 42 per cent and cardiology 32 per cent.[50] A review of 7836 neurological patients at the Charing Cross Hospital found that 26 per cent were medically unexplained, while a further 4 per cent were diagnosed as suffering from 'conversion hysteria'.[51]

The dilemma of how to respond to patients with *medically unexplained symptoms* has contributed to the emergence of many new and contested diseases or syndromes, such as irritable bowel syndrome, fibromyalgia, chronic or post-viral fatigue syndrome, repetitive strain injury, and whiplash. These syndromes share a common absence of observable physical pathology and rely on the subjective reports of the patient. Somatic syndromes of this kind account for 20 per cent of primary care consultations in the UK[52] and 35 per cent of new medical outpatient referrals.[53]

The new syndromes are contested because although their diagnosis is based on self-reported symptoms which cannot be verified by reference to observable abnormalities in the body, patients insist that their condition is essentially organic rather than psycho-social. Sufferers have formed pressure groups to promote understanding of their illnesses, to lobby for further research to discover the elusive physiological basis of the disease and to provide support for fellow sufferers.[54] Social scientists have documented the activities of such groups as well as researching the experiences of sufferers.[55,56] A common pattern emerges from these accounts: the onset of disabling symptoms, followed by the doctor's failure to arrive at a physical diagnosis, endless referrals and ineffective treatments, often concluding with the suggestion that the problem is psychological rather than organic. Importantly, it is often the doctor's invalidation of the patient's illness claim, rather than the failure to provide a satisfactory treatment or cure that causes most dissatisfaction.[57] The career of such patients and the agenda of pressure groups representing them is not primarily about the pursuit of a cure, but the demand for recognition of the physical character of their illness; described as the 'search for legitimacy', or more graphically as the 'pilgrimage of pain'.[58]

Wessely et al.[59] argue that *functional somatic syndromes* of this kind have much in common in terms of case definition, symptoms, and patient characteristics including sex, outlook and response to treatment, and should be treated as a single (and by implication psycho-social) syndrome rather than several different forms of organic disease. However, syndrome debunkers face an uphill struggle. While the scientific method can demonstrate that no evidence has been found that a particular syndrome is organic rather than psycho-social, it cannot claim that no such evidence will be found in the future. Even when the available evidence appears to have put the question beyond reasonable doubt, for example, in Andrew Malleson's compelling critique of the whiplash epidemic, popular support often keeps the phenomenon alive.[60]

Whatever their origin it would be wrong to conclude that medically unexplained symptoms are necessarily less disabling and distressing than those for which physical pathology can be found. Carson et al.[61] in their prospective cohort study of 300 neurological referrals found that one-third had symptoms that were not explained by organic disease, however, patients with lower organicity ratings reported more pain and disability than those with observable physical disease. Other studies comparing non-specific and specific symptoms support this. Patients attending hospital with the medically unexplained irritable bowel syndrome exhibit greater distress and disorder than those with inflammatory bowel disease,[62] and chronic fatigue syndrome is often more disabling than heart failure.[63]

Faced by the subjective experience of suffering, and mindful of the dangers of invalidating the patient, general practitioners often feel obliged to accept the illness claims of their patients even when no evidence of pathology can be found. A recent study of sickness certification found that general practitioners had great difficulty performing their role as gatekeeper to sickness benefits and that 'in practice most operate a "sick certificate on demand" system'.[64] This has contributed to an epidemic of sickness and incapacity. The number of recipients of Incapacity Benefit (the main welfare benefit paid to the long-term ill or disabled) rose from 700,000 in 1979 to 2.6 million in 1995 (although the increase has been stable since then), with much of this increase attributable to non-specific illnesses, particularly chronic pain and mental health problems such as work stress.[65] The economic costs are considerable, with the number of working days lost to work stress alone now greater than the number lost to strike action during the 'winter of discontent' in 1978–9.[66] However, the costs are not purely financial. There is evidence to suggest that uptake of Incapacity Benefit may have a disabling effect, with mental and physical health deteriorating rather than improving over time; after a year on Incapacity Benefit recipients are more likely to die or retire on benefit than they are to return to work. Focusing on the capacity for work, rather than encouraging the adoption of a disabled identity not only brings economic savings, it is often also in the best interests of the patient.

The epidemic of incapacity has raised the problem of how illness behaviour should be governed, for example, the government's recent reform of the Incapacity

Benefit system is a response to this imperative.[67] Piloted in the *Pathways to Work* programme, the proposed measures aim to draw a distinction between those with severe physical impairment who are incapable of work and those with less severe illnesses who, with appropriate support and incentives, could return to work. Ironically, the epidemic that such measures address has its origins in the changes to the discourse of health associated with the incorporation by government of the New Public Health and its active promotion of patient-centred practice. The redefinition and expansion of the categories of health and wellbeing; the heightened sense of vulnerability generated by countless health scares and healthy lifestyle campaigns; the erosion of evidence of physical pathology as the basis of diagnosis, and its replacement by the patient's subjective account of symptoms; have fuelled an epidemic of illness behaviour which has little basis in disease. The following section explores this contradiction.

Governing illness behaviour

The changes that have occurred in the discourse of health over the last 40 years are contradictory. The broader definition of health and the growing acceptance of the social models have expanded the medical domain into new areas of everyday life, but the authority of the medical profession to police the boundary between sickness and health has been eroded as the adoption of patient-centred medical practice has undermined the doctor's ability to reject the illness claims made by the patient. To understand this paradox we must look more closely at how medical sociologists have conceptualised the relationship between medicine and social control. We begin by going back to 1950s America and Talcott Parsons's exploration of the normative function of medical practice.[68]

The sick role

Parsons's account of the sick role is not meant to describe illness behaviour and medical practice, but to explain how medicine overcomes the disruption caused by illness and returns the patient to 'normal' functioning. The doctor presides over this process regulating access to the sick role by validating or rejecting illness claims, and prescribing treatments which will restore health. For Parsons, the main function of medical practice is the control of deviant behaviour and the maintenance of social order, not through overt coercion, but by moral consensus over the obligations and entitlements that the sick role entails, which are:

- suspension of some of the duties associated with normal social roles, for example, paid employment, housework, looking after dependents;
- abdication of moral responsibility for the illness, that is, the patient is not blamed for becoming ill;
- duty to leave the sick role as soon as possible and return to normal social functioning;
- obligation to seek professional medical care.

For Parsons, these entitlements and obligations stem from shared values which emphasise normal role performance and the desire to overcome illness and return to health. The possibility that patients might engage in prolonged illness behaviour in order to gain exemption from 'the rigours of everyday life' is recognised by Parsons, but only as an 'unconscious motivation'.[69] The role of the doctor does not entail policing the behaviour of the patient, but assisting in a shared project of overcoming illness.

Parsons has been criticised for assuming that this process of normalisation is consensual. Freidson has argued that the doctor–patient relationship is often characterised by conflict and negotiation rather than an unquestioning acceptance of medical authority.[70] The emergence of contested diseases, such as fibromyalgia or RSI has heightened this tension. The doctor's legitimation of entry to the sick role is not a purely technical exercise based upon evidence of pathology, but a socially negotiated process in which the patient's subjective account of the illness may prevail. In Parsons's model, medical knowledge gives the doctor an easily exercised authority over the patient who simply acquiesces in clinical decision making; however, as Hardey has pointed out, this power relationship is now in doubt.[71] Not only has the balance of power in the doctor–patient relationship changed, but the emergence of patient-centered practice and initiatives such as the expert patient programme reflect a broader questioning of medical authority which Parsons does not address.

Parsons's emphasis upon the return to normal social functioning does not fit well with chronic or terminal illness. Parsons responded to this criticism by suggesting that successful management or adaptation is equivalent to the restoration of health.[72] This revision extends the explanatory range of the sick role to include a different set of endpoints, but it sheds little light on the epidemic of medically unexplained (and usually chronic) illnesses. In Parsons's later formulation the emphasis is still on the return to social functioning, but with the added recognition that the physical reality of disease may limit the achievement of that objective. What Parsons fails to recognise or predict is the extent to which the objective of returning to normal social functioning would be eroded by changes in the discourse of health.

Parsons assumed that the urge to recover from illness and return to optimum role functioning is universal, but this leaves him unable to explain the well-documented variations in illness behaviour between men and women, different social classes and ethnic groups. The value ascribed to the duties and entitlements of the sick role varies between social groups, reflecting differences in socialisation.[73]

The socialist critique of Parsons's formulation suggests that the sick role merely represents the articulation of middle-class values of commitment to work and personal responsibility, and that rather than undesirable deviance illness is a legitimate form of social dissent.[74,75] The proposition that entry to the sick role may serve as a means of expressing alienation or dissatisfaction with the world of work is compelling. The rapid rise in the number of incapacity benefit recipients in the decade up to 1995 mirrored the decline in unemployment benefit rates as the government tightened access to the latter, and the work stress phenomenon overtly links unhappiness at work to sick role entry. However, as a form of dissent illness has little to offer, for example, the identity of 'work stress victim' is essentially passive and while many have presented it as a critique of capitalist production relations and an imperative towards job redesign,[76] in practical terms the response from employers has been minimal and therapeutic, comprising for example, the introduction of stress management and counselling interventions, rather than radical changes in job control or demands. Rather than the vanguard of social change, the ill represent agency and political will at its most diminished.

Parsons's account of the sick role may fit well with the Protestant work ethic, serving to reintegrate workers into the production process, but where this cannot be achieved long-term incapacity offers an identity which is *almost* as functional in terms of maintaining social order, providing a sink for surplus labour and channelling those who cannot or will not work into the politically safe domain of health services and welfare benefits. If Parsons is to be criticised it is for overlooking the function of long-term incapacity for the maintenance of social order, rather than for failing to recognise dissent.

Both Parsons and his socialist critics over-estimate the role of curative medicine in maintaining social order. The duties and obligations of the sick role have been eroded since Parsons first articulated them in the 1950s. The doctor no longer stands as an effective gate-keeper to the sick role. Patient-centred medicine and the critique of the bio-medical model have displaced evidence of physical pathology as the entry requirement for the sick role in favour of the subjective claims of the patient. Sick notes are given on demand and a host of new and medically unexplained syndromes are at hand to avoid invalidating the patients claims. The duty to seek professional care may still formally exist, but the obligation to comply with doctor's orders has been weakened by notions of mutuality and concordance.[77,78]

These changes have substantially weakened what Parsons saw as the main moral obligation of the sick role – the duty to recover from illness and return to normal social functioning at the earliest opportunity. Rather than stigmatising long-term illness and insisting on a hasty return to health, modern medicine has presided over a rapid expansion of illness behaviour, mainly in the form of non-specific psycho-social conditions. These changes amount to a fundamental decline in the moral authority of curative medicine. Medicine still cures people and still returns them to full social functioning, but the critique of bio-medicine and the valorisation of new illness identities have robbed this process of its moral force – as a medium of social control curative medicine is a very leaky bucket indeed.

The moral authority of curative medicine, described in Parsons's theory of the sick role, may be declining, but the discourse of health is still embroiled in social regulation, albeit in a different form. The imperative of health is no longer exercised through the obligations and duties of the sick role, but through a new emphasis on the pursuit of 'wellbeing'. For Parsons, health was normative and illness was a form of deviance which medicine aimed to repair. The new discourse of health has not so much inverted the relationship between health and illness so much as clouded the distinction between the two. The belief that health is the normal state of human existence, from which illness is a departure, has been replaced by a heightened sense of vulnerability and risk in which the boundary between sickness and health is less clearly defined and more easily crossed. Bio-medicine has had considerable success in overcoming physical pathology, but improvements in objective measures of health status have not led to an enhanced sense of durability. Rather than feeling that we have triumphed over disease we increasingly feel that health is a fragile state easily shattered by the wrong lifestyle choices or social experiences.[79] In Parsons's conception of the sick role, the patient was not responsible for his illness; disease was viewed as an aspect of nature that was external to human consciousness and, therefore, beyond personal control. This belief that disease is an external threat to humanity that must be defeated by curative medicine is rapidly being replaced by the anthropogenic view that ill health is man made, either through personal behaviour such as smoking, bad diet, lack of exercise, or through the actions of others who expose the individual to, for example, environmental pollution, stressful workplaces, or unhealthy school meals.

This approach has been described as 'victim blaming',[80] but this is inaccurate as ill health is seen as the product of a wider network of social relations and not just the choices of the individual. More accurately the anthropogenic view of illness could be referred to as 'human blaming'. Moreover, the notion of 'blaming' implies a *post-hoc* moral judgement ascribed to the ill; however, the vague concept of wellbeing inverts the relationship between illness and blame, it is not so much that the sick are blamed for their ill health, as that the disease-free are judged according to their efforts in pursuing the elusive goal of wellbeing. Smokers, the over-weight, heavy drinkers and the sexually promiscuous are increasingly stigmatised, not just for the health problems they have, but also for their 'high-risk' behaviour which may (or may not) lead to health problems in the future.[81] Where Parsons's sick role viewed the patient as a blameless victim whose duty was to return to health as soon as possible, moral authority is now exercised through the healthcare system by pathologising the behaviour of those who do not follow the strict dictates of 'healthy living'.

A consequence of this transition is to shift health from a normative state enjoyed by most people, most of the time, though threatened by degenerative disease and external pathogens, into an elusive and poorly specified aspiration. If health is conflated with happiness and wellbeing, then any problematic aspect of everyday life, whether it is bullying in the playground, abusive relationships in the home or stress at work, becomes a legitimate grounds for therapeutic intervention. Not only does this expand the domain of health intervention to almost everyone, it also gives rise to a new sense of personhood, defined by a heightened sense of vulnerability and a tendency to suspend the duties and expectations of normal social functioning in response to the challenges of everyday life.

The normalisation of illness behaviour has eroded the moral imperative to return to normal social functioning which Parsons described as the main obligation of the sick role. The emphasis has shifted from the struggle to overcome physical pathology and recover from the limitations imposed by disease, towards endless exhortation to reduce risk factors and adopt healthy lifestyles, in order to avoid becoming ill in the first place. This strategy, coupled with the other changes in the discourse of health described earlier, has contributed to a continual increase in forms of illness behaviour which appear to have little basis in physical pathology. It seems that the more effort is put into identifying risk factors and promoting healthy lifestyles, the greater the increase in subjective health problems. The response to the epidemic of subjective health problems has not been to reassert the sovereignty of physical pathology as the entry requirement for the sick role, but the adoption of a psychotherapeutic approach which effectively medicalises the management of subjectivity and the negotiation of everyday life.[82]

Sociologists have long claimed that medicine is a form of social control.[83] The evidence presented in this chapter supports the view that health policy and the healthcare system are implicated in social regulation, impelling people to moderate risky behaviour and expanding the remit of the therapeutic state to oversee the pursuit of wellbeing. However, this form of social control is substantially different to the coercive powers of the state as they are exercised in, for example the military, or the criminal justice system. Changes in the discourse of health have deepened the state's footprint in everyday life, but instances of direct coercion are rare. It would also be a mistake to assume that there is a hidden agenda being pursued which serves the interests of a political or professional elite. Some professional groups, such as those engaged in health promotion or counselling, have expanded, but the resources they command and their formal powers are limited. Fitzpatrick is correct in referring to a 'tyranny of health', in which ever increasing areas of everyday life are governed by the imperative of wellbeing,[84] but it is important to recognise that this is a tyranny which is largely free from direct coercion, which confers little benefit on those who wield it, and which seems likely to further inflate the epidemic of illness behaviour that it seeks to reduce.

Understanding Mrs Lancaster's injury

This chapter opened with an account of Mrs Lancaster's stress-related injury. Three questions were posed which can now be revisited: Why are problems of everyday life, such as coping with the demands of a new job, experienced as health problems which can lead to sick leave or early retirement on medical grounds? Is injury or illness fundamentally a description of physical changes in the body, or is it a way of behaving in the world which can exist independently of physical pathology? And, if illness resides in behaviour rather than organic disease then who is responsible for its occurrence; the person exhibiting it or the external agents or circumstances that provoked it?

The discourse of health has broadened beyond physical disease, to include emotional states and social circumstances which previous generations would not have recognised as health problems. The concept of work stress originates in this expansion. Although stress has physical correlates, including the production of hormones which prepare the body for action, it is not a disease as such, but a way of making sense of experiences which can stimulate illness behaviour even in the absence of disease. Work stress differs from a broken leg because it is grounded in the meaning ascribed to experiences by the individual, rather than in unconscious damage to the body.

Mrs Lancaster's entry to the sick role was possible because of the emergence of a patient-centred approach which prioritises subjective reports of symptoms over physical evidence of pathology. Diagnosis of work stress does not depend upon blood tests or X-rays, but on the patient's claim that they are suffering from a condition caused by their experiences at work. Although work stress is a form of illness behaviour grounded in the subjectivity of the individual, the new discourse of health locates its origins in external social determinants. Although this avoids stigmatising the individual, it also constructs her as a passive victim rather than as an active subject. This may shift responsibility from the employee to the employer, but it comes at a high price. In return for time off work or financial compensation, the work stress victim must enter the sick role, and endure all this entails in terms of limitations on role performance and life chances.

Changes in the discourse of health provide a medicalised web of meaning through which experiences at work can be made sense of. Mrs Lancaster's 'injury' is a response to this, but it is by no means inevitable. Many people experience problems at work, including a heavy workload, or antagonistic relations with managers or customers, but not everyone makes sense of such problems by reference to the discourse of health. Previous generations had different explanatory frameworks grounded in economics, politics, or industrial relations. Historical change may have left these explanations without practical strategies for achieving change, but the first step in developing new ways of addressing the problems of everyday life is to reject the passive identity conferred by the sick role and embrace that of the resilient social agent.

Conclusion

This chapter has explored the ways in which our changing ideas about what constitutes health and illness have influenced behaviour. Most dramatically, the broadening of definitions of illness, coupled with the promotion of a heightened sense of mental and physical vulnerability, have fuelled a rapid increase in illness behaviour much of which is medically unexplained, while the focus on patient-centred practice has diluted the capacity of the medical profession to police the boundary between sickness and health.

Discussion topics

- What is the difference between disease and illness?
- If no physiological evidence of disease can be found to explain a patient's symptoms, in what sense is their claimed illness legitimate? Discuss with reference to chronic fatigue syndrome or repetitive strain injury.
- What effect have recent changes in the discourse of health had on the social control of illness behaviour?

Further reading

Arksey, H. (1998) *RSI and the Experts*. London: UCL Press.

A case study which explores the tensions between sufferers of this new 'disease' and the medical profession.

Fitzpatrick, M. (2001) *The Tyranny of Health: Doctors and the Regulation of Lifestyle*. London: Routledge.

A detailed critique of the New Public Health from a libertarian standpoint.

Wainwright, D. and Calnan, M. (2002) *Work Stress: The Making of a Modern Epidemic*. Buckingham: Open University Press.

A critique of the scientific literature on work stress and an account of the historical and sociological factors that gave rise to the epidemic.

Young, J.T. (2004) Illness behaviour: a selective review and synthesis. *Sociology of Health & Illness*, 26(1): 1–31.

An excellent account of the development of this key concept including recent formulations of it.

References

1   The *Independent*, 6 July 1999, p. 6.
2   The *Guardian*, 7 July 1999.
3   Porter, R. (1997) *The Greatest Benefit to Mankind: A Medical History of Humanity from Antiquity to the Present*. London: Harper Collins.
4   Sapolsky, R.M. (1991) Poverty's remains. *The Sciences* 31: 8–10.
5   Littlewood, R. and Lipsedge, M. (1982) *Aliens and Alienists: Ethnic Minorities and Psychiatry*. Harmondsworth: Penguin.
6   Miles, A. (1991) *Women, Health and Medicine*. Milton Keynes: Open University Press.
7   McWhinney, I.R. (1997) *A Textbook of Family Medicine (2nd edn)*. Oxford: Oxford University Press.
8   Mechanic, D. and Volkart, E. (1961) Stress, illness behaviour and the sick role. *American Sociological Review*, 26: 52.
9   Mechanic, D. (1978) *Medical Sociology (2nd edn)*. New York: The Free Press.
10 Zborowski, M. (1952) Cultural components in responses to pain. *Journal of Social Issues*, 8: 16–30.
11 Zborowski, M. (1952) ibid., p. 28.
12 Freidson, E. (1970) Dilemmas in the doctor–patient relationship. In: C. Cox and A. Mead (eds), *A Sociology of Medical Practice*. London: Collier MacMillan.
13 Koos, E. (1954) *The Health of Regionville: What People Thought and Did About It*. New York: Columbia University Press.
14 Verbrugge, L. (1986) From sneezes to adieux: stages of health for American men and women. *Social Science and Medicine*, 22(11): 1195–212.
15 Calnan, M. (1987) *Health & Illness: The Lay Perspective*. London: Tavistock.
16 Blaxter, M. and Paterson, L. (1982) *Mothers and Daughters: A Three Generation Study of Health Attitudes and Behaviour*. London: Heinemann.
17 Young, J.T. (2004) Illness behaviour: a selective review and synthesis. *Sociology of Health and Illness*, 26(1): 1–31.
18 Giddens, A. (1979) *Central Problems in Social Theory*. London: Macmillan.
19 Frankl, V.E. (2004) (1946) *Man's Search for Meaning*. London: Rider & Co.
20 Archer, M.S. (2003) *Structure, Agency and the Internal Conversation*. Cambridge: Cambridge University Press.
21 Calnan, M. and Gabe, J. (1991) Recent developments in general practice: a sociological analysis. In J. Gabe, M. Calnan, and M. Bury (eds), *The Sociology of the Health Service*. London: Routledge 61.
22 Wainwright, D. and Calnan, M. (2002) *Work Stress: The Making of a Modern Epidemic*. Buckingham: Open University Press.
23 Mills, C. Wright (1970) *The Sociological Imagination*. Harmondsworth: Penguin.
24 MacKenzie, M.D. (1946) The World Health Organisation. *British Medical Journal*, 21 September: 428–30.
25 Klein, R. (2000) *The New Politics of the NHS (4th edn)* London: Prentice Hall.

26 Fitzpatrick, M. (2001) *The Tyranny of Health: Doctors and the Regulation of Lifestyle*. London: Routledge.

27 Ashton, J. and Seymour, H. (1988) *The New Public Health*. Milton Keynes: Open University Press.

28 Townsend, P. and Davidson, N. (eds) (1988) *Inequalities in Health. The Black Report & The Health Divide*. Harmondsworth: Penguin.

29 Department of Health (1988) *Short-term Prediction of HIV Infection and Aids in England and Wales (Cox Report)*. London: HMSO.

30 Fitzpatrick, M. (2001) ibid.

31 Acheson, D. (1988) *Public Health in England: The Report of the Committee of Inquiry into the Future Development of the Public Health Function*, CM289. London: HMSO.

32 Skrabanek, P. (1994) *The Death of Humane Medicine and the Rise of Coercive Healthism*. London: Social Affairs Unit.

33 Department of Health (July 1999) *Saving Lives: Our Healthier Nation* (White Paper). London: The Stationery Office.

34 Fitzpatrick, M. (2001) ibid.

35 Furedi, F. (2004) *Therapy Culture: Cultivating Vulnerability in an Uncertain Age*. London: Routledge.

36 Baeza, J.I. (2005) *Restructuring the Medical Profession: The Intraprofessional Relations of GPs and Hospital Consultants*. Buckingham: Open University Press.

37 Jefferys, M. and Sachs, H. (1983) *Rethinking General Practice: Dilemmas in Primary Medical Care*. London: Tavistock.

38 Armstrong, D. (1979) The emancipation of biographical medicine. *Social Science and Medicine*, 13A: 1–8.

39 Pearse, I.H. and Crocker, L. (1943) *The Peckham Experiment*. London: Allen & Unwin.

40 Williams, S. and Calnan, M. (1994) Perspectives on prevention: the views of general practitioners. *Sociology of Health and Illness*, 16: 372–93.

41 Balint, M. (1964) *The Doctor, His Patient and the Illness*. London: Pitman Medical.

42 Williams, S.J. and Bendelow, G. (1998) *The Lived Body: Sociological Themes, Embodied Issues*. London: Routledge.

43 Smith, B.H. (2001) Chronic pain: a challenge for primary care. *British Medical Journal*, 51: 524–6.

44 Kleinman, A. (1988) *The Illness Narratives: Suffering, Healing and the Human Condition*. New York: Basic Books, p. 10.

45 Stimson, G.V. (1974) Obeying the doctor's orders: a view from the other side. *Social Science and Medicine*, 8: 97–104.

46 Royal Pharmaceutical Society of Great Britain (1997) *From Compliance to Concordance: Towards Shared Goals in Medicine Taking*. London: RPS.

47 Clarke, J.N. (2000) The search for legitimacy and the 'expertization' of the lay person: the case of Chronic Fatigue Syndrome. *Social Work in Health Care*, 30: 73–93.

48 Wainwright, D., Calnan, M., O'Neill, C., Winterbottom, A. and Watkins, C. (2006) When pain in the arm is 'all in the head': the management of medically unexplained suffering in general practice. *Health, Risk & Society*, 8(1): 71–88.

49 Kroenke, K. and Mangelsdorff, A.D. (1989) Common symptoms in ambulatory care: incidence, evaluation, therapy and outcome. *American Journal of Medicine*, 86: 262–6.

50 Hamilton, J., Campos, R. and Creed, F. (1996) Anxiety, depression and the management of medically unexplained symptoms in medical clinics. *Journal of the Royal College of Physicians*, 30: 18–20.

51 Perkin, G.D. (1989) An analysis of 7836 successive new outpatient referrals. *Journal of Neurology, Neurosurgery and Psychiatry*, 52: 447–8.

52 Peveler, R., Kilkenny, L. and Kinmonth, A.L. (1997) Medically unexplained physical symptoms in primary care: a comparison of self-report screening questionnaires and clinical opinion. *Journal of Psychosomatic Research*, 42(3) 245–52.

53 Hamilton, J., Campos, R. and Creed, F. (1996) ibid.

54 Arksey, H. (1998) *RSI and the Experts*. London: UCL Press.

55 Carke, J.N. (2000) ibid.

56 Reid, J., Ewan, C. and Lowy, E. (1991) Pilgrimage of pain: the illness experiences of women with repetition strain injury and the search for credibility. *Social Science and Medicine*, 32: 601–12.

57 Deale, A. and Wessely, S. (2001) Patients perceptions of medical care in chronic fatigue syndrome. *Social Science and Medicine*, 52: 1859–64.

58 Reid, J. Ewan, C. and Lowy, E. (1991) ibid.

59 Wessely, S. Nimnuan, C. and Sharpe, M. (1999) Functional somatic syndromes: one or many? *The Lancet*, 354: 936–9.

60 Malleson, A. (2002) *Whiplash and other useful illnesses*. London: McGill-Queen's University Press.

61 Carson, A.J., Ringbauer, B., Stone, J., McKenzie, L., Warlow, C. and Sharpe, M. (2000) Do medically unexplained symptoms matter? A prospective cohort study of 300 new referrals to neurology outpatient clinics. *Journal of Neurology, Neurosurgery and Psychiatry*, 68: 207–10.

62 Walker, E.A., Roy Byrne, P.P., Katon, W.J., Li, L., Amos, D. and Jiranek, G. (1990) Psychiatric illness and irritable bowel syndrome: A comparison with inflammatory bowel disease. *American Journal of Psychiatry*, 147: 1656–61.

63 Komaroff, A.L., Fagioli, L.R., Doolittle, T.H., Gandek, B., Gleit, M.A., Guerriero, R.T. et al. (1996) Health status in patients with chronic fatigue syndrome and in general population and in disease control groups. *American Journal of Medicine*, 101: 281–90.

64 Hussey, S., Hoddinott, P., Wilson, P., Dowel, J. and Barbour, R. (2003) Sickness certification in the United Kingdom: qualitative study of views of general practitioners in Scotland. *British Medical Journal*, 328: 88–91.

65 Waddel, G. and Aylward, M. (2005) *The Scientific and Conceptual Basis of Incapacity Benefits*. London: TSO.

66 Durodie, B. (2005) *The Concept Of Risk*. Paper commissioned by The Nuffield Trust for the UK Global Health Programme.

67 Secretary of State for Work and Pensions (January 2006) *A New Deal for Welfare: Empowering People to Work*, Cm 6730. London: Department for Work and Pensions.

68 Parsons, T. (1951) *The Social System*. New York: Free Press.

69 Young, J.T. (2004) ibid.

70 Freidson, E. (1960) Client control and medical practice. *American Journal of Sociology*, 65: 374–82.

71 Hardey, M. (1999) Doctor in the house: the internet as a source of lay health knowledge and the challenge to expertise. *Sociology of Health and Illness*, 21(6): 820–35.

72 Parsons, T. (1975) The sick role and the role of the physician reconsidered. *Millbank Memorial Fund Quarterly,* 53: 257–78.

73 Young, J.T. (2004) ibid.

74 Waitzkin, H. and Waterman, B. (1974) *The Exploitation of Illness in Capitalist Society.* Indianapolis, IN: Bobbs-Merrill.

75 Birenbaum, A. (1984) *Health Care and Society.* New Jersey: Allenheld and Osmun.

76 Karasek, R. and Theorell, T. (1990) *Healthy Work: Stress, Productivity and the Reconstruction of Working Life.* New York: Monthly Review Press.

77 Szasz, T. and Hollender, M. (1956) A contribution to the philosophy of medicine: the basic models of the doctor-patient relationship. *Journal of the American Medical Association,* 97: 585–8.

78 Stimson, G.V. (1974) Obeying the doctor's orders: a view from the other side. *Social Science and Medicine,* 8: 97–104.

79 Furedi, F. (2004) *Therapy Culture: Cultivating Vulnerability in an Uncertain Age.* London: Routledge.

80 Crawford, R. (1977) You are dangerous to your health: the ideology and politics of victim-blaming. *International Journal of Health Services,* 7(4): 663–80.

81 Peterson, A. (1997) Risk, governance and the new public health. In A. Petersen and R. Bunton (eds), *Foucault, Health and Medicine.* London: Routledge.

82 Furedi, F. (2004) ibid.

83 Zola, I. (1972) Medicine as an institution of social control. *The Sociological Review,* November: 487–504.

84 Fitzpatrick, M. (2001) ibid.

6

Medicalisation in a Therapy Culture

Frank Furedi

- Medicalisation refers to the process by which everyday experiences become redefined as health problems.
- Early formulations of the medicalisation thesis viewed it as a conscious strategy adopted by the medical profession to extend its power and influence.
- The diminution of professional dominance, coupled with the emergence of new forms of medicalisation which are largely independent of the profession has led to medicalisation being reformulated as a broader cultural dynamic.
- Where an earlier generation bridled against the intrusion of medicine into everyday life, there is now a growing tendency to normalise illness and seek therapeutic intervention as a means of defining and validating identity.

From sex to food, from aspirins to clothes, from driving your car to riding the surf, it seems that under certain conditions, or in combination with certain other substances or activities or if done too much or too little, virtually anything can lead to certain medical problems. I at least have been convinced that living is injurious to health.

Irving Zola, 1972.

Medicalisation is the process through which areas of everyday life have come under the purview of medical authority. Through this process a growing range of normal experiences have become redefined as health issues that require medical intervention. Medicalisation can also be seen as an attempt to provide an alternative interpretation to problems of existence. Many issues that were the subject of community deliberation, or the responsibility of religious leaders, families, or the individuals concerned, are increasingly represented as matters for the health professional. With the domain of emotions becoming a central site for professional intervention, medicalisation has steadily expanded in recent decades.

Medicalisation is one of those rare sociological terms that have entered the vocabulary of everyday life. Although the medical establishment was one of the original targets of this thesis, doctors now denounce the threat of 'creeping medicalisation'. The *British Medical Journal*, the prestigious publication of the UK medical establishment published a special issue on medicalisation in 2002.[1] The growing usage of this sociological concept is underpinned by its resonance with contemporary cultural processes. Conditions such as cancer, obesity and AIDS, along with drugs such Viagra and Prozac, have as many cultural significances as they have medical connotations. The cultural significance of the idiom of health has steadily expanded during the past three decades. Terms like 'sexual health' or 'healthy lifestyle' signify normative and moral statements about the world. Advice on health has become institutionalised and may have displaced the role previously assumed by moral injunction.

Since its emergence in the late 1960s and early 1970s, medicalisation theory appears to have been validated by subsequent developments. This period has seen a steady expansion of medical boundaries as more and more individual and social experiences are framed in medical terms as an illness or disorder. The promotion and celebration of health as the paramount value of western society have encouraged people to interpret a growing range of human activities through the vocabulary of medicine. Illness categories are used to make sense of routine problems of existence. Shyness, apprehension of failure, the inability to focus on tasks, promiscuity, childlessness are just some of the problems that come with a medical diagnosis. Conditions that hitherto were confined to children, for example, Attention Deficit Hyperactivity Disorder, are now diagnosed in adults. And men are now claiming to suffer from illnesses that were until recently regarded as specifically women's conditions, such as post-natal depression and the menopause. They are represented as 'conditions' that people experience rather than the outcome of the way people behave. According to one study in recent decades the meaning of obesity has been transformed 'from being the product of something that individuals *do* to something they *experience*'.[2] The ever-widening definition of illness has been paralleled by the steady growth in expenditure on health. Not surprisingly, the health industry has been an important beneficiary of, and contributor to, the medicalisation process.

Medicalisation and professional power

The medicalisation thesis emerged as a critique of medical professionalism, and specifically of medical power. It represented a reaction against rationality, expert knowledge and the biomedical model of health. Frequently the exercise of this power was portrayed as a form of social control – particularly the control of women's bodies or of behaviour that failed to conform to prevailing norms. For many of its influential proponents, medicalisation was associated with the conscious pursuit of medical interest through establishing hegemony in defining and managing health and illness. The metaphor of 'medical imperialism' was used to represent the idea of the expansionary ambition of a predatory profession.

Freidson in his *Profession of Medicine*[3] took the view that the exercise of medical authority often contradicted the interest of the public. Others too argued that medicine tended to disempower the patient and that it did more harm than good. Illich[4] took the view that the medical profession undermined people's capacity to look after themselves and forced patients to become dependent on professionals. 'The medical establishment has become a major threat to health', claimed Illich.[5] Michel Foucault argued that the ascendancy of professional power of doctors led to their convergence around the *medical gaze*, through which the sick are represented as objects for surveillance and technical intervention.[6] An early critic of medicalisation expressed the fear that dependency on the authority of the medical expert would lead to the 'medicalisation of life' where the status of 'the patient' could become the norm.[7]

Concerns were also raised about the medicalisation of deviant behaviour. At various times crime, alcoholism, mental illness, homosexuality, child and drug abuse have been endowed with a medical label. It was suggested that such medical labels serve as a form of veiled condemnation of groups whose behaviour was labelled as a form of illness.[8] However, it was also evident that medicalisation did not simply focus on deviant behaviour, but also sought to give meaning to important dimensions of everyday normal experience. Pregnancy, birth, death, ageing, menopause, anger, shyness and anxiety are some of the ordinary aspects of life that have been presented as medical issues requiring professional management. Feminist writers claimed that women constituted a prime target of this process. They argued that reproduction, pregnancy and childbirth had been transformed and medicalised by the medical profession. In this way women were dispossessed of their historically dominant role in managing the reproductive process. The shift from a midwife-managed home birth to a male specialist overseeing it in a hospital has been interpreted as the consolidation of male medical domination.[9]

Medicalisation was sometimes represented as an expansive process that threatened to transform the day-to-day problem of existence into an issue of health. From this perspective medicalisation is seamlessly bound up with the changing cultural valuation of health and safety. According to Zola, since health has become a 'paramount value' in society the sphere of medicine inevitably assumes significance as an institution of social control.[10]

The end of professional dominance

The strength of the medicalisation thesis was its ability to draw attention to the tendency to reinterpret problems of existence as medical conditions. The weakness of early formulations of the thesis was the association of the process of medicalisation with the promotion of narrow professional interest. As one of the early critics of this argument stated:

> in light of the multi-institutional and the cultural significance of health, illness, and medicine in all societies it is both illogical and unlikely to believe that the current process of medicalisation in American society has been engineered and maintained primarily by one group, namely, the physicians.[11]

The early focus on professional interest tended to distract contributors from exploring the cultural influences that assisted the expansion of medicalisation. It is difficult to see how a project driven by narrow professional interest succeeded in gaining such a powerful influence over people's imagination. From a sociological perspective it is evident that concern with health must resonate with cultural forces if it is to gain influence over people's lives.

That the medical profession often acts according to its distinct interest is not in doubt. That the exercise of this professional interest – particularly the maintenance of a gate-keeping role to the regulation and management of health – can create distortions and conflict with the public good is also confirmed by experience. However, it is far from evident how the exercise of professional interest can account for the powerful cultural currents that promote medicalisation. That is why from the outset the thesis of medical imperialism has been questioned by medical sociologists such as Phil Strong.[12] Others pointed out that in many instances, such as the management of alcoholism, the medical profession played only a marginal role in controlling and defining an illness.

In the 1980s, the radical critique of professional power gained legitimacy from the ascendancy of a wider mood of cultural suspicion of expertise and professional authority. Furthermore, this radical critique of professional authority was complemented by market-oriented and managerially inspired attacks on medical autonomy. One outcome of this process has been the growth of a trend towards the diminishing of individual clinical judgment through the institutionalisation of clinical governance frameworks and other forms of regulation. One important consequence of this process has been the widely noted decline in status of the medical profession. Studies of the 'loss of legitimacy' of the medical profession in the USA point to the ascendancy of corporations, the pharmaceutical industry and of managed care.[13,14] In line with this development contributions on medicalisation tended to attach less significance to the role of the profession in the promotion of this process.

Throughout western societies the medical profession faces a crisis of authority and confidence. There is now a growing literature that points to the displacement of medical authority by the deprofessionalisation and deskilling of the medical profession. Some contributors point to the growing pressure on the medical profession from the expansion of state regulation and managerial surveillance. Suspicion towards doctors is further reinforced by the growth of alternative authorities such as complementary medicine, patients' groups and the professionalisation of other occupational groups such as nurses. It is evident that the cultural process of medicalisation is not mediated only through the medical professions. Psychologists, mentors, life coaches, herbalists, parenting coaches and bewildering variety of counsellors are more than happy to offer their diagnoses of any illness afflicting the individual. The institutionalisation of litigation has also played an important role in the erosion of professional authority. The medical profession is facing a challenge to its authority and claims to professionalism from patients' and self-help groups, environmental health movements, holistic and alternative critics of biomedicine, advocacy groups promoting lay expertise or consumerism. This challenge from below is encouraged by the cultural turn against expertise and authority. The medical profession is also facing pressure from above. The managerial revolution in health care and the growing tendency of the state to police professional life has contributed to the decline of medical authority.

Today the growth of medicalisation coexists with the diminishing of professional authority and power. That is why in the twenty-first century, the argument that represents the profession as the main driver of medicalisation is rarely put forward with conviction. Not surprisingly the emphasis of the medicalisation thesis has shifted to account for new developments and the changing cultural norms through which health and illness are experienced. In particular, the focus of the thesis on the assertion of professional medical power has given way to a variety of other issues. Peter Conrad, one of the early theorists of medicalisation accounts for this shift of emphasis on the grounds that although 'doctors are still gatekeepers for medical treatment', their 'role has become more subordinate in the expansion or contraction of medicalisation'.[15] Conrad claims that in the past 'the medical profession and the expansion of medical jurisdiction was a prime mover for medicalization'. However, he claims that since the 1980s 'pharmaceutical companies have become a major player in medicalization', which along with managed care, the transformation of patients into consumers, and biotechnology are the 'engines that drive medicalisation in western societies'.[16]

In recent years the role of the pharmaceutical industry has been associated with the medicalisation process by a number of contributors. Carpiano's study of the way that erectile dysfunction came to be medicalised through Viagra reinforces Conrad's conclusion.[17] Moynihan and Cassels argue that the aggressive marketing of new drugs by pharmaceutical companies is often carried out through the construction of new medical conditions. They illustrate their argument by pointing to newly invented conditions, such as Female Sexual Dysfunction. This is one of those conditions for which a drug exists before there is any clarity about how to define the disease.[18]

While the pharmaceutical industry plays an important role in the construction of new illnesses, it is far too simplistic to represent it as the engine that drives the process of medicalisation. It is likely that the very idea of a consciously driven process needs to be rethought. Institutions like the medical profession in the past or the pharmaceutical industry in the present may reap some of the benefits of medicalisation but the process itself is an outcome of a cultural dynamic rather than of the intentional behaviour of individuals. As Verweij noted, 'the involvement of medical professions may be a consequence; it is not necessarily the engine in medicalization processes'. It 'is first and foremost a conceptual phenomenon: a change in discourse and a concurrent change of the way people see and understand certain things in their lives'.[19]

Medicalisation from below

The thesis of professional imperialism is not the only idea put forward by the early theorists of medicalisation that appears to be inconsistent with the experience today. It is increasingly difficult to sustain the claim made by the early proponents of the medicalisation thesis, that the patient is the passive target of medical control. While the model of the top-down medicalisation process may have corresponded to the experience of the late 1960s and early 1970s, it is difficult to argue this case today. The past two decades have seen the rise of the 'expert patient' and advocacy organisations and self-help groups that are devoted to contesting medical authority. These movements contest the status of medical diagnosis and of expertise. They assign lay experience a privileged status and demand institutional, scientific and cultural affirmation for their representation of the constitution of illness. In contrast to the expectation of some of the critics of the medical profession, these groups do not threaten or diminish the power of the process of medicalisation. On the contrary, it can be argued that today one of the more powerful influences on the trend towards medicalisation is the transformation of the docile patient into a consumer or an active patient in search of a diagnosis.

The shift from medicalisation from above to below is reflected in the growing influence of the Foucauldian approach to this subject. Unlike the early theories that stressed the importance of professional power and interest, proponents of the Foucauldian approach stress the importance of medical discourse in the construction of identity. From this standpoint the construction of the self involves the individual in the active processes of contesting and internalising elements of medical discourse. This celebration of the active subject of medicalisation creates ambiguities in the way that the process is conceptualised. Medicalisation is represented both as a potentially coercive form of social control and a creative force in the construction of new identities, or the promotion of what some have called lay reskilling. Unlike the traditional form of medicalisation identified by the early theorists, bottom-up medicalisation is sometimes portrayed in a more positive light in the current literature. According to one account, 'for some people medicalisation provides meaning, understanding and legitimation of their experience of impairment'.[20]

However it is conceptualised, medicalisation from below represents a challenge to the thesis that it is a form of social control that is one dimensionally imposed from above. According to one account, 'in some situations lay people may initiate or collude with the medicalisation of their distress in order to access the benefits and support they need to manage their symptoms of everyday life'. In such circumstances 'the undue emphasis in the analysis of medicalisation on a unilateral imposition of meaning on patients' bodies will not help solve the current dilemma'.[21]

The medicalisation of everyday life

Whether or not medicalisation involves the pursuit of professional interest, the intentional promotion of professional power is not its main driving force. Rather its growth has been underwritten by socio-cultural processes that continually throw up a demand for medical definitions to make sense of existential problems. Above all, the demand for medicalisation is generated by cultural changes that inflate the sense of individuation and of powerlessness. These changes, such as the thinning-out of community attachments and the decline of systems of moral meaning, were reinforced in the 1980s by the demise of social solidarity. Since then, the individuation of social experience has heightened the sense of personal vulnerability, creating further opportunities for health-related issues to encroach into the realm of social experience.

The experience of the 1980s represents a distinct phase in the history of medicalisation. Throughout the past two centuries there have been numerous struggles against attempts to medicalise certain forms of behaviour and people. During the 1960s, the anti-psychiatry movement was in the forefront of questioning various claims that defined people as mentally ill. In the 1970s, the campaign against the diseasing of same-sex relationships succeeded in demedicalising homosexuality. Until the 1980s, the medicalisation of women's experiences, particularly in the domain of reproduction, was fiercely contested. Feminist and other critics challenged the medicalisation of childbirth and of abortion. In contrast, today leading feminist voices such as Naomi Wolf are in the forefront of promoting the medicalisation of childbirth through popularising the diagnosis of post-natal depression. 'Postpartum depression affects 400,000 mothers per year in the USA', argues Wolf.[22] Recent attempts to medicalise female behaviour – pre-menstrual syndrome, battered women's syndrome, new mother's syndrome – are now rarely challenged.

Since the 1980s, opposition to medicalisation has been minimal. This period has also seen an unprecedented expansion in the medicalisation of social experience. This is the era of dyslexia, sex addiction, attention deficit disorder, social phobia and co-dependency. Increasingly, it is not professional bodies but grass-roots campaigners who are in the forefront of demanding a medical label to describe their condition. Organisations demanding recognition for ME or fibromyalgia are highly critical of doctors who are reluctant to recognise their claim for a medical label. Campaigners promoting the cause of Gulf War Syndrome reject as an insult the suggestion that they are not suffering from a physically based illness. Advocacy groups promoting medical recognition of chronic fatigue syndrome have sought to raise money to finance 'the discovery of diagnostic markers and treatments that would legitimize and indeed, medicalize the constellation of symptoms they experience'.[23]

In an interesting study, Conrad and Potter explore how the medicalised concept of Attention Deficit Hyperactivity Disorder (ADHD), which was once diagnosed as a children's condition expanded to the world of the adult. The study emphasises that medicalisation is 'usually a product of collective action' rather than a result of 'medical imperialism. In this case it has led to the inclusion of an entire group of people who were not originally part of the diagnosis of hyperactive children. It points to the role of 'diagnostic advocacy' of social movements in expanding the boundaries of medicalisation.[24] They note that in contrast to the experience of ADHD with children, this condition among adults tends to be self-diagnosed. From their overview of this experience, the authors contend that 'the lay promotion of adult ADHD and the predominance of self-diagnosis contradict some of the basic premises of labelling theory' which ' suggests a fundamental conflict between social control agents and putative deviants'.[25] In this case, rather than serving as a form of social control, medicalisation is 'embraced and promoted by the people who receive it'. This case also illustrates a trend towards 'diagnostic expansion'; a process whereby one 'legitimated medical category can beget others'.[26]

The activities of patients' groups and of movements critical of expertise, technology and professionalism are often interpreted as representing a trend towards the demedicalisation of society. The influence accorded to holistic health and lay expertise is sometimes represented as symptomatic of a trend away from medicalisation. However, a closer inspection of the activities of these movements indicates that their target is not medicalisation *per se* but the professional authority of the physician. Lupton writes of the 'contradiction and naivities inherent in the calls for "demedicalisation" since the exhortation for self-care can move medical and health concerns into every corner of life'.[27] As Williams hints, lay self-help groups are involved in a 'peculiarly medicalised form of demedicalisation'.[28] Consequently it is far more useful to conceptualise the activities of patient groups and advocacy organisations as representing a challenge to the professional authority of the doctor than to the medicalisation of social experience. The confusion of demedicalisation with *deprofessionalisation* distracts attention from one of the defining features of contemporary times – which is that most significant developments that shape the process of contemporary medicalisation are generated outside the institution of medicine.

Socio-cultural developments

From its inception proponents of the medicalisation thesis took the view that this development was bound up with the imperative of social control. Some of the early pioneers, Zola (1972) and Freidson (1970), took the view that medicine had assumed many of the functions of social regulation previously associated with religious and legal institutions. According to Zola's path-breaking analysis, medicine was 'becoming the new repository of the truth, the place where absolute and often final judgements are made by supposedly morally neutral and objective experts'. He added that the expanding influence of the institution of medicine was 'largely an insidious and often undramatic phenomenon accomplished by "medicalizing"much of daily living, by making medicine and the labels "healthy" and "ill" *relevant* to an ever increasing part of human existence'.[29] This 'undramatic' phenomenon can be seen as part of the process of cultural transmission whereby a growing range of human experiences are represented as subjects that are interpreted through the prism of health and illness.

The growing demand for a diagnosis is linked to wider socio-cultural developments. The objective of a healthy life-style is promoted through a network of public institutions. According to one account, it is the representation of wellbeing as a fundamental right that encourages individuals in society to become preoccupied with their health. This sentiment leads to the idealisation of 'positive health' – a valuation of wellbeing in all spheres of existence: 'The concept of positive health is responsible for the steadily increasing tendency to medicalisation because it favours the involvement of medicine not only in the diseases but also in the psychological, social and ethical illnesses'.[30] That is why 'the push for medical legitimation' may 'never in fact have been greater' than today.[31]

Health promotion has acquired an obsessive character. It has also been embraced by governments committed to establishing points of contact with an otherwise disengaged public. One of the implicit messages transmitted through campaigns against obesity and other 'unhealthy' life styles is that health is not something that people have, but something that can only be achieved through effort and work. From this perspective, health acquires an elusive quality and illness is transformed into a normal state of existence. Perversely the paramount value attached to health has the effect of normalising illness. At the same time, as Azzone contends, the line that used to divide an illness from disease also becomes blurred. He argues that 'the conceptual and practical blending of disease and illness favours the medicalisation of the patient's personal experience and behaviour'.[32] It can be argued that the constant preoccupation with health can have the perverse outcome of undermining one's 'feelings of confidence and security regarding one's health and well being'. In circumstances where people are instructed to 'constantly anticipate threats against their health', confidence in one's state of health may be undermined.[33]

One of the disturbing developments associated with the process of medicalisation has been the confusion that accompanies debates about the meaning of illness and health. Consequently, the line that divides health from illness has become increasingly blurred. In previous times, the sociology of medicine was based on the premise that the sick role was a temporary one and that illness was an undesirable state and not a normal state of being. In his major contribution to the subject, Talcott Parsons assumed that the relationship between a doctor and patient was underpinned by a shared positive valuation of health and a negative valuation of illness.[34] Yet today, definitions of illness are highly contested and a negative valuation of illness is itself a subject of controversy. 'For some, the patient career may be a permanent way of life, with a self-supporting network of friends, activities, doctors and treatments', writes Showalter.[35] Being ill can now constitute a defining feature of an individual's identity. The positive valuation of certain forms of illness even enjoys a degree of cultural affirmation. One study of women's experiences of fibromyalgia claims that the illness can create intimacy and kinship. It suggests that this experience 'provides one with an opportunity to recognise oneself'.[36] Another study of cancer-related identity speculates about how this illness can be a 'potentially positive experience.[37] In popular culture identities associated with an illness are often portrayed in a positive light. In some cases individuals suffering from Asperger's Syndrome and other types of disability are portrayed as possessing special positive qualities that their healthy counterparts lack.

Confusion about the meaning of illness has encouraged conflicting valuations of medical conditions. Some illnesses have been harnessed to the project of identity construction. The medicalisation of social experience has encouraged some to regard their illness as not something they suffer from, but as the defining feature of who they are. Some groups and individuals claim to positively value being deaf or blind. Literature produced by some patient groups enthuses about the positive experience with their illness, claiming that it helped construct a sense of intimacy, kinship and community. Newspaper columns written by individuals living with cancer examine the virtues of their condition. This valorisation of the 'positive' features of illness calls into question the original conceptualisation of the sick role. According to its original formulation, the sick role is interpreted as a temporary episode. If, as today, the sick role is experienced as an affirmation of identity, it is likely to assume a more durable character. Terms like 'cancer survivor' or 'recovering alcoholic' testify to a growing tendency to represent illness as constituting a long-term influence on identity.

Of course most people who are ill endeavour to get well as fast as possible. Most people seek health and are not likely to reconcile themselves to being ill. But confusion about the meaning of health and illness, and the development of illness-based identities constitute a continuous invitation to the expansion of medicalisation. It indicates that the expansion of the boundary of medicine has the unexpected consequence of contributing to the normalisation of illness.

In its original form the medicalisation thesis highlighted the process through which social deviance was frequently recast in a medical form. Activities that were traditionally interpreted as immoral or socially undesirable were redefined as symptoms of illness. The focus on the medicalisation of deviance has been systematically elaborated in the contributions of Peter Conrad. He presented this dimension of medicalisation as an important form of social control.[38] But what happens when illness is not represented as a form of deviance? One interesting outcome of medicalisation is the normalisation of illness. As the state of illness assumes a normal form, it becomes more and more difficult to interpret it as a form of deviance. Insofar as there is a relationship between medicalisation and deviance it is not focused on a specific condition but on the refusal of the individual to seek help. Help seeking is invariably represented as a marker of individual maturity. In contrast, individuals who refuse to seek help are condemned for their irresponsible behaviour.[39]

Influence of culture

People's perceptions of health and illness are shaped by the particular account that their culture offers about how they are expected to cope with life and about the nature of human potential. Individuals make sense of their experience through reflecting on their specific circumstances and in line with the expectations transmitted through prevailing cultural norms. People have no inner desire to perceive themselves as ill. However, powerful cultural signals provide the public with a ready-made medicalised interpretation of their troubles. And once the diagnosis of illness is systematically offered as an interpretative guide for making sense of distress, people are far more likely to perceive themselves as ill. That is why, despite the steady advance in public health and medicine, an increasing section of society define themselves as ill, or suffering from a long-term illness or disability. In the UK, government officials have been at a loss to account for the fact that between 1985 and 1996 there has been a 40 per cent increase in the number of people who consider themselves disabled. The authors of the survey have concluded that the difference between the 1985 and 1996 figures 'appear too large to be explained by a real increase in the prevalence of disability' but find it difficult to explain why more and more people are so enthusiastic about embracing the disabled label.[40]

The readiness with which the pathologisation of human behaviour is embraced indicates that the medicalisation of life has become an accomplished fact. The demand for a medical diagnosis is fuelled by confusion about individual perceptions of the self. At a time of existential insecurity, a medical diagnosis at least has the virtue of definition. A disease explains an individual's behaviour and it even helps confer a sense of identity. The medicalisation of everyday life allows individuals to make sense of their predicament and gain a sense of identity.

The search for identity: demand for diagnosis

The growth of identities that are embodied in a medical condition creates a demand on doctors to validate their patients' accounts of their experiences. In this relationship medical authority remains intact but the imperative towards medicalisation is initiated from below. Doctors who fear that affirming their patients' diagnoses may have negative consequences sometimes become uncomfortable accomplices in the process of medicalisation. Some doctors who have resisted the pressure to endow a patient's complaint with a medical label have faced intense pressure and hostility. For example, Chronic Fatigue Syndrome activists in the USA have reacted with fury against doctors who question this diagnosis, accusing them of an act comparable to Holocaust denial. Some illness groups justify their existence on the ground that their claims are not legitimised by medical authority. Successful advocacy by The Fibromyalgia Association, and other like-minded groups, that the condition's sufferers were ignored led the World Health Organisation (WHO) to incorporate fibromyalgia into its International Classification of Diseases. The medicalisation of a condition through an officially designated label is seen to give legitimacy to those living with this illness. In turn, those who suffer from this condition claim that the legitimation accorded their diagnosis has helped them gain meaning from it.

The campaign to gain recognition for the diagnosis of fibromyalgia demonstrates that in contemporary times the demand for medicalisation comes from below. According to an important study of this search for symptom meaning 'a key element in the process of medicalization is the coming together of sufferers within self-help communities to translate their individual experiences of distress into a shared expression of illness'.[41] This search for an illness identity is an important theme in contemporary claims making. Indeed, for some people the search for a medical diagnosis has assumed the character of a crusade. In the European Union, an organisation titled 'Rare Disorder Alliance' has been launched to gain prompt diagnosis for people suffering from rare disorders.[42]

Under pressure from advocacy and parents' support groups, a growing number of British doctors now diagnose and treat hyperactivity in children. Those who promote 'awareness' of this illness, claim that 'identification of the problem is useful in itself' because 'any harm done by labelling' is outweighed by the benefits to self-esteem.[43] Medical labels are eagerly sought by some parents for their children. So hyperactive children are now 'considered to have an illness rather than to be disruptive, disobedient, overactive problem children'.[44] Parents are actually relieved when they 'discover' that their child has got some medical problem and is not responsible for his or her behaviour. 'I got my best Christmas present a few days before the big day this year', wrote a mother in *The Times*. She was referring to the wonderful news that her son was diagnosed as dyslexic and was therefore clearly not lazy, as she previously feared.[45] Until this diagnosis, school reports characterised the child as 'easily distracted' and 'occasionally disruptive'. As a victim of dyslexia the child will no longer be subject to official disapproval. Instead, the child can now expect recognition and moral support.

Henrietta Rose, who has written a book – *A Gift in Disguise* – about her difficult experience of bringing up a son with severe learning disability, is still disappointed that her son Tom was never diagnosed with a named condition. She claims, that as a result she 'missed the opportunity to start mourning' the loss of her dreams and expectations'.[46] This importance attached to recognition means that often parents look for a named condition, even when their children do not have a serious disability like Tom. A medical label eases the difficulty of dealing with problem behaviour. There is evidence in Britain that both teachers and parents collude in the popularisation of the learning disabled classification in schools. At a time of existential insecurity, a medical diagnosis at least has the virtue of definition. A disease explains an individual's behaviour and it even helps confer a sense of identity. The medicalisation of everyday life allows individuals to make sense of their predicament and gain moral sympathy. Klasen argues that 'parents tended to experience medicalization and labelling as important aspects of validation and legitimation of their experience, which gave them a sense of control and led to improved parent-child relationships'. From this perspective the demand for the medicalisation of children appears as a positive act of empowerement. That is why Klasen warns doctors who are reluctant to medicalise that they can 'deligitimate parents' experience, this increasing their suffering'.[47]

An important study into the experiences of women claiming to suffer from Repetition Strain Injury stresses the significance that the claimants attached to gaining recognition for their plight. The authors of the study report that the 'issue which dominates many of the women's accounts of their illness is that of credibility'. The study describes the naming of their condition as Repetition Strain Injury as the initiation of a 'pilgrimage of pain', the seeking of external validation of their condition. 'Women spoke of their symptoms as if the diagnosis was a matter of faith rather than medicine, and their pilgrimage centered on finding other believers who may be able to offer help', observed the authors.[48] This search for sympathy and recognition and validation through a medical label motivates many of the illness groups that are mushrooming throughout society.

The association of identity with a medical condition encourages the expansion of medicalisation and also creates a demand for new forms of treatment. It has given a major boost to the medicalisation of sexual behaviour and of sexual pleasure. Sex has been recast as an important dimension of a healthy lifestyle and people are encouraged to 'seek treatment' if they do not feel sexually gratified. The term 'sexual health' indicates that the conduct of intimate life has also become dominated by the medical imperative. The medicalisation of sexual pleasure illustrates how treatment supported identities help fuel the market for health. The market for health is influenced by the construction of a demand from below which is encouraged and cultivated by institutions of health promotion and the pharmaceutical industry. In this process doctors still play a role, albeit a modest one.

The experience of the past three decades indicates that the medicalisation process is driven and shaped by influences that are distinct from the activities of the medical profession. Moreover the expansion of medical boundaries may well conflict with the interests of the medical profession and may even have contributed to its demise. Traditionally, medicalisation has been seen as a means by which doctors increased their power over other associated practitioners, such as midwives and herbalists, and over patients. Today, medicalisation needs to be understood in a different context. Strangely, one of the most significant by-products of medicalisation is the end of the professional dominance of the doctor. In a society that privileges the discourse of health and wellbeing, vested interests in medical matters extend far beyond doctors. Indeed, those who were once in the centre of the picture now seem to be pushed out of the frame.

The colonisation of everyday life

The process of medicalisation is not confined to diagnosing problems linked to the body. In cultural terms it involves exporting the ideas of illness and disease beyond the body to make sense of conditions and experiences that are distinctly cultural and social. One of the most important ways in which medicalisation has evolved during the second half of the twentieth century has been through 'discovering' diseases that are non-physical and are to do with emotional problems. Increasingly, psychological problems to do with stress, rage, trauma, low self-esteem or addiction provide a medical label for interpreting virtually every human experience. The growth of a cultural sensibility oriented towards therapy offers medicalisation a vast territory for further expansion. Strictly speaking, the process that we are describing can be more accurately expressed as that of *psychologisation* rather than medicalisation. However, given the wide spread usage of the latter we shall use it to describe the process through which personal problems are recast as medical or psychological conditions.

The ascendancy of therapeutic culture should not be confused with the growing influence that therapy exercises over people's lives. Growing interest in therapy should be conceptualised as a cultural phenomenon rather than as a clinical technique. As the sociologist Robert Bellah put it, it is 'a way of thinking rather than as a way of curing psychic disorder'.[49] A culture becomes therapeutic when this form of thinking expands from informing the relationship between the individual and therapist to shaping public perceptions about a variety of issues. At that point it ceases to be a clinical technique and becomes an instrument for the management of subjectivity.

A culture encompasses a system of beliefs about the meaning of life and offers a vocabulary through which we can make sense of an individual's relationship to society. Cultural representations of this relationship are underpinned by perceptions of what constitutes the individual. Every culture offers a statement about human nature and insights into the potential and limitations of human action. Therapeutic culture today offers a distinct view about the nature of human beings. It tends to regard people's emotional state as peculiarly problematic and at the same time as defining their identity. As a result, therapeutic culture regards the management of emotion as the most effective way of guiding individual and collective behaviour. The management of emotion is invariably conducted through its medicalisation.

Professionalisation

The process of medicalisation has been inseparable from that of professionalisation. A diagnosis is a prelude to its professional management. As James Chriss writes, 'professional organizations whether organized around medicine, law, business, social science, or the burgeoning array of helping professions – always seek to expand the range of objects and phenomena to which their members' expertise may arguably be applied'.[50] This expansive dynamic is in part driven by economic expedience and by the opportunities created by the modern state. As Dineen argues, the Psychology Industry is 'first and foremost a business, intent on selling its services and expanding its market'.[51] Since the nineteenth century, professionals have been remarkably successful in creating a demand for their services. Lasch claims that 'the new professions themselves invented many of the needs they claimed to satisfy'. He adds that 'they played on public fears of disorder and disease, adopted a deliberately mystifying jargon, ridiculed popular traditions of self-help as backward and unscientific, and in this way created or intensified (not without opposition) a demand for their own services'.[52] However, the pursuit of professional self-interest cannot, on its own, account for the all pervasive tendency to medicalise social experience. As Hochschild notes, 'the significance of the growth of new therapies cannot be dismissed by the argument that they are simply a way of extending jobs in the service sector by creating new needs'. The question remains, 'why *these* needs?'.[53]

These needs – including the demand for medicalisation – are generated by cultural changes that inflate the sense of individuation and of powerlessness. These changes – the thinning-out of community attachments, the decline of systems of moral meaning – were reinforced in the 1980s by the demise of politics and social solidarity. The individuation of social experience has heightened the sense of personal vulnerability creating further opportunities for the market to encroach into the realm of social experience.[54] According to the British psychologist David Smail, 'there was a positive explosion in the expansion of the therapy and counselling industry in Britain'. This explosion was made possible by an all-pervasive cultural tendency to redefine personal difficulty as a pathology requiring professional management. Smail notes that as part of this process 'the market was extended in several new directions and "counselling" – previously considered a minority practice of doubtful validity – suddenly became the self-evident necessary antidote to occasions of distress which up till then people had just had to muddle through as best they could'. Smail gives the examples of disaster counselling and the development of the concept of Post-traumatic Stress Disorder as examples of the 'extension of the frontiers of the market into previously non-commercial territory of ordinary social intercourse'.[55]

The readiness with which the pathologisation of human behaviour is embraced indicates that the medicalisation of life has become an accomplished fact. New opportunities exist for the professionalisation of human behaviour and in turn professional intervention creates a greater demand for medicalising the problems of day-to-day living. The provision of counselling advice – no matter how sound and common sensical – further diminishes the capacity of people to negotiate the problems they encounter. The problem is not that professional advice is always misguided, but that it short-circuits the process through which people can learn how to deal with problems through their own experience. Intuition and insight gained from personal experience is continually compromised by professional knowledge. This has the unintentional consequence of estranging people from their own feelings and instincts since such reactions require the affirmation of the expert. In such circumstances people's capacity to handle relationships and to have confidence in their relationships diminishes further.[56] This only creates new opportunities for professional intervention in everyday life.

Professional intervention unleashes a process whereby the dependency of the individual on the expert becomes increasingly more systematic. The mediation of experience by the professional has the effect of distancing people from one another, thereby fragmenting the network of relationships further still. Although the process of fragmentation is bound up with the process of modernity, its professionally mediated form is a relatively recent development. Moreover, the mediation of experience through the professional alters the very character of human relationships. The mediation of experience undermines the organic links that sustain relationships. The problem is removed from its real-life context and is reconstituted as an object of professional management. As mediators of experience, professionals cannot help but alter the relationship between people. Couples who carry out intimate communication with their counsellor end up communicating to one another in a different way. Parents who are discovering their children's problems through discussions with the expert become distracted from developing forms of communication with their children that are the outcome of spontaneous interaction. Interdependence between people vies with dependence on the professional, thereby complicating the conduct of relationships.

Probably the most significant legacy of professionalisation is that it encourages the *formalisation* of relationships. A seminal study carried out by Robert Bellah and his colleagues draws attention to the way in which therapeutic attitudes distance American people from their 'social roles, relations, and practices'. Instead of friends, neighbours, elders and the many informal roles that have no name, we have peers, mentors, appraisers, life-style gurus, personal trainers and a whole army of counsellors. Even intimate relationships have become subject to the influence of contract-like procedures. Bellah is not so much concerned about the danger of professional domination of personal life. He fears 'that too much of the purely contractual structure of economic and bureaucratic world is becoming an ideological model for personal life'. He concludes that 'the prevalence of contractual intimacy and procedural co-operation, carried over from boardroom to bedroom and back again, is what threatens to obscure the ideals of both personal virtue and public good'.[57]

It is the ability of therapy to reinterpret social experience into personal meaning that motivates many to seek professional support. However, the attempt to contain the psychic effects of rationalisation through therapy has the perverse consequence of expanding rationalisation into the domain of intimate relationships. Through the professionalisation of everyday life, formal procedures are introduced into the realm of personal relations. The formalisation of relationships imports ideas of self-interest, calculation and mistrust into the realm of intimacy. Its effect is to render relationships impersonal – thereby creating an even greater demand for the promise of a personalised remedy offered by therapeutics.

From the standpoint of the therapeutic imperative it is not so much a profession but the professionalisation of human life that encourages the promotion of medicalisation. The medicalisation of human experience is not so much about rendering people ill as about casting them into the role of powerless and helpless individuals.

Conclusion

Medicalisation has been a central concept in medical sociology since the early 1970s. Early conceptions focused on the efforts of the medical profession to promote its status and power at the expense of the passive patient. Today medicalisation refers to a much broader cultural process than professional self-promotion. Instead the impetus for medicalisation comes from below, as medicalised frames of reference are invoked to explain and give meaning to ever wider areas of everyday life. At the same time, the therapeutic relationship through which the power of the medical profession was exercised over patients has been duplicated in countless other relationships, formalising them and rendering them impersonal.

Discussion topics

- Has the medicalisation of life become an 'accomplished fact'?
- Is medicalisation best characterised as a conscious strategy adopted by a vested interest in order to extend its power, or, as the product of a more diffuse cultural dynamic?
- What are the consequences of translating the troubles of everyday life into health problems?

Further reading

Azzone, C.F. (1998) *Medicine from Art to Science.* Amsterdam: IOS Press.

Azzone provides a useful historical account about the transformation of western medicine and its status. This book provides an interesting background to contemporary debates on the legitimacy of medical knowledge.

Conrad, P. (2005) The shifting engines of medicalization. *Journal of Health and Social Behavior*, 46(1): 4–5.

Peter Conrad's work on medicalisation has influenced sociological thinking on this subject. This article provides useful insight into the changing influences on the process of medicalisation.

Furedi, F. (2004) *Therapy Culture: Cultivating Vulnerability in an Uncertain Age.* London: Routledge.

This book explores the way that medicalisation has shifted its focus towards mental health and the emotions. Its emphasis is on the cultural influences that shape perceptions of individual wellbeing.

Williams, S.J. (2001) Sociological imperialism and the profession of medicine revisited: where are we now? *Sociology of Health and Illness*, 23(2): 135–58.

A useful update on the tensions between medical sociology and its subject matter, first addressed by Phil Strong (see further reading to Chapter 1), with particular emphasis on medicalisation.

References

1   *British Medical Journal* (13 April 2002) 324.
2   Chang, V.W. and Christakis, N.A. (2002) Medical modelling of obesity: a transition from action to experience in a 20th century American medical textbook. *Sociology of Health and Illness*, 24(2): 151.
3   Freidson, E. (1970) *Profession of Medicine*. New York: Dodd Mead.
4   Illich, I. (1975) *Limits to Medicine: The Expropriation of Health*. London: Calder & Boyars.
5   Illich, I., Zola, I.K., McKnight, J., Caplan, J. and Shaiken, H. (1977) *Disabling Professions*. London: Marion Boyars, p. 11.
6   Foucault, M. (1963) *The Birth of the Clinic: An Archaeology of Medical Perception*. London: Tavistock.
7   Zola, I.K. (1972/1978) ibid.
8   Conrad, P. (1992) Medicalization and Social Control. *Annual Review of Sociology*, 18: 209–32.
9   Oakley, A. (1984) The *Captured Womb: A History of the Medical Care of Pregnant Women*. Oxford: Blackwell.
10 Zola, I.K. ibid.
11 Fox, R.C. (1977) The medicalization and demedicalization of American society. *Daedalus*, 106(1): 14.
12 Strong, P.M. (1979) Sociological imperialism and the profession of medicine: a critical examination of the thesis of medical imperialism. *Social Science and Medicine*, 13A(2): 199–215.
13 Stevens, R. (2001) Public roles for the medical profession in the United States: beyond theories of decline and fall. *The Milbank Quarterly*, 79(3): 327.
14 Schlesinger, M. (2002) A loss of faith: the sources of rescued political legitimacy for the American medical profession. *The Milbank Quarterly*, 80(2): 185.
15 Conrad, P. (2005) The shifting engines of medicalization. *Journal of Health and Social Behavior*, 46(1): 3.
16 Conrad, P. (2005) ibid., pp 4–5.
17 Carpiano, R.M. (2001) Passive medicalisation: the case of Viagra and erectile dysfunction. *Sociological Spectrum*, 21(3): 441–50.
18 Moynihan, R. and Cassels, A. (2005) *Selling Sickness: How Drug Companies Are Turning Us All Into Patients*. New York: Allen & Unwin, p. 176.
19 Verweij, M. (1999) Medicalization as a moral problem for preventive medicine. *Bioethics*, 13(2): 92.
20 Mulvany, J. (2001) Disability, impairment or illness? The relevance of the social model of disability to the study of mental disorder. In J. Busfield (ed.), *Rethinking the Sociology of Mental Health*. Oxford: Blackwell, p. 52.

21 Busby, H., Williams, G. and Rogers, A. (1997) Bodies of knowledge: lay and biomedical understandings of musculosketal disorders. In M.A. Elston (ed.), *The Sociology of Medical Science and Technology.* Oxford: Blackwell, pp. 93–4.

22 Wolf, N. (2001) *Misconceptions, Truths, Lies and the Unexpected on the Journey to Motherhood.* London: Chatto and Windus, p. 185.

23 Clarke, J. (2000) The search for legitimacy and the 'expertization' of the lay person: the case of chronic fatigue syndrome. *Social Work in Health Care,* 30(3): 74.

24 Conrad, P. and Potter, D. (2000) From hyperactive children to ADHD adults: observations on the expansion of medical categories. *Social Problems,* 47(4): 558.

25 Conrad, P. and Potter, D. (2000) ibid.

26 Conrad, P. and Potter, D. (2000) ibid.

27 Lupton, D. (1997) Foucault and medicalisation critique. In A. Petersen and R. Bunton (eds) *Foucault, Health and Medicine.* London: Routledge, p. 107.

28 Williams, S.J. (2001) Sociological imperialism and the profession of medicine revisited: where are we now? *Sociology of Health and Illness,* 23(2): 146.

29 Zola, I.K. (1972/1978) ibid.

30 Azzone, C.F. (1998) *Medicine from Art to Science.* Amsterdam: IOS Press, p. 152.

31 Williams, S.J. (2001) ibid., p. 146.

32 Azzone, C.F. (1998) ibid., p. 148.

33 Verweij, M. (1999) Medicalization as a moral problem for preventive medicine. *Bioethics,* 13(2): 97.

34 Parsons, T. (1951) *The Social System.* New York: Free Press.

35 Showalter, E. (1997) *Hystories: Hysterical Epidemic and Modern Culture.* London: Picador, p. 19.

36 Sodberg, S., Lundman, B. and Norberg, A. (1999) Struggling for dignity: the meaning of women's experience of living with fibromyaglia. *Qualitative Health Research,* 9(5): 584.

37 Zebrack, B. (2000) Cancer survivor identity and quality of life. *Cancer Practice,* 8(5): 241.

38 Conrad, P. (1992) ibid., p. 216.

39 Furedi, F. (2004) *Therapy Culture: Cultivating Vulnerability in an Uncertain Age.* London: Routledge, p. 35.

40 Furedi, F. (2004) ibid., p. 113.

41 Barker, K. (2002) Self-help literature and the making of an illness identity: the case of fibromyalgia syndrome. *Social Problems,* 49(3): 295.

42 See the web site of this organisation: www.eurodis.org

43 Taylor, E. and Hemsley, R. (1995) Treating hyperkinetic disorders in childhood. *British Medical Journal,* 310: 1617–18.

44 Conrad, P. (1975) The discovery of hyperkinesis: notes on the medicalisation of deviant behaviour. *Social Problems,* 23: 18.

45 *The Times,* 26 December 1997.

46 Cited in the *Guardian,* 30 September 1998.

47 Klasen, H. (2000) A name, what's in a name? The medicalization of hyperactivity revisited. *Harvard Review of Psychiatry* 7(6): 334.

48 Reid, J., Ewan, C. and Lowy, E. (1991) Pilgrimage of pain: the illness experiences of women with repetition strain injury and the search for credibility. *Social Science Medicine,* 32(5): 609–11.

49 Bellah, R., Madsen, R., Sullivan, W. et al. (1996) *Habits of the Heart: Individualism and Commitment in American Life*. Berkeley, CA: University of California Press, p. 203.

50 Chriss, J.J. (ed.) (1999) *Counselling and the Therapeutic State*. New York: Aldine de Gruyter, p. 6.

51 Dineen, T. (1999) *Manufacturing Victims: What the Psychology Industry Is Doing to People*. Toronto: Robert Davies, p. 244.

52 Lasch, C. (1979) *The Culture of Narcissism: American Life in an Age of Diminishing Expectations*. New York: Warner Books, p. 383.

53 Hochschild, A.R. (1983) *The Managed Heart: The Commercialization of Human Feeling*. Berkeley, CA: University of California Press, p. 192.

54 Furedi, F. (2004) ibid.

55 Smail, D. (2001) *The Origins of Unhappiness: A New Understanding of Personal Distress*. London: Robinson.

56 How this process informs the parent and child relationship is discussed in Furedi (2001).

57 Bellah, R., Madsen, R., Sullivan, W. et al. (1996) ibid., p. 127.

7

The 'Feminisation' of Health

Ellie Lee and Elizabeth Frayn

- The past 20 years have seen the emergence of a new discourse of health, at the centre of which is the idea that 'prevention is better than cure'.
- Contemporary health concerns are often 'gendered'. The emergence of campaigns about 'men's health' is a notable development of recent years.
- There is a striking contrast between feminist constructions of the problem of women's health in the 1970s, and the contemporary problem of gender and health.
- In the context of the new discourse of health, 'masculinity' has come to be defined as a barrier to health. 'Feminine' attitudes such as a willingness to consider oneself vulnerable and 'at risk', and to seek help have, in turn, been validated as desirable characteristics for both men and women.
- Contemporary gendered health concerns have much less to do with evidence-based developments in science and medicine, than with developments in the spheres of politics and society.
- The practical outcome of the feminization of health is that men as well as women may become more anxious and worried about their health, for little discernable benefit.

Masculinity is among the more significant risk factors associated with men's illness. [It] is not only a risk factor in disease etiology but it is also among the most significant barriers to men developing a consciousness about health and illness.

Michael Kimmel, 1995

A cursory examination of contemporary health concerns suggests that gender is significant for their construction. The idea set out above, for example, that 'masculinity' is a key 'risk factor' associated with ill health, is now widely held. The notion that a 'male' outlook on life is 'unhealthy', and is likely associated with the development of disease, has become commonplace.

It is not only the specialist and academic literature that discusses the significance of gender for ill health in this way. Cultural support is offered to the notion that 'masculine' attitudes and behaviours are unhealthy and undesirable, and by implication 'feminine' ones preferable. 'Binge drinking' for example, is often typified in the media by images of drunk, young women staggering through town centres. Headlines draw attention to the idea that a part of this problem of alcohol consumption today is the way in which young women are 'copying' the 'masculine', 'risky' behaviour typical of young men. An unfortunate outcome of greater sex equality, this approach suggests, is that women are becoming more 'unhealthy', as they are prone to behave in a way that is more 'male' than that of women in the past.

What should we make of this way of thinking about health and illness? How and why has 'masculinity' come to be stigmatised as unhealthy? It is useful to think of the 'gendering' of health concerns as part of the overall process this volume seeks to investigate. This is the emergence of what has been termed the 'new paradigm' of health and health care,[1] or, the new discourse of health (See chapters 1 and 5), and it draws upon the following set of related precepts:

- *Ill health is caused by attitudinal and behavioural factors.* Disease in contemporary society, it is claimed, results from the way society is organised, and in 'unhealthy' behaviour and attitudes that emerge as a result.
- *The emphasis of health care should shift from cure to prevention.* Health care, it is argued, needs to become more focused on health promotion programmes that encourage people who are not yet ill to be alert to the need to 'choose health' and modify their behaviour accordingly.
- *The meaning of 'health' should be redefined.* 'Health', it is suggested, should no longer be an assumed state of normality, and become instead a state of being that all apparently healthy individuals should ideally actively pursue in the course of their everyday life, through changing their behaviour.
- *Illness is best considered less an occasional aberration from normality to be addressed when it occurs, more a constant risk facing everybody.* It is suggested that an awareness of the risk of becoming ill is a useful outlook for people to have, since this requires us to engage as a matter of course in minimising our likelihood of becoming ill.

In sociological terms, this approach to health and illness can be thought of as one that makes *identity* central to definitions of health and ill health, as the following extract explains:

> Rather than simply being told how to act, or being treated by medical interventions when ill, people are being increasingly induced to monitor their own health and are being instilled with healthy attitudes. The control of health must therefore come from *within* the person.[2]

The new discourse of health brings with it an important socio-cultural process. It is *the life inside* the individual that is deemed in need of modification, since in order for health to be attained, change must take place *within the person*. In other words, it is *attitudes and emotions*, how individuals *think and feel*, that become the focus for the pursuit of health; or in the words of Kimmel, it is a 'consciousness of health and illness' that is considered to be the ideal mindset, and those who seek to improve health must find ways to develop this consciousness in others.[3]

In contemporary society, the means through which modification of behaviour, attitudes and feelings is now enacted is legion. There are many different ways in which people are being encouraged to monitor and control health from 'within the person'. Confronting and changing 'masculinity' can be considered one of them, however, and the primary purpose of this chapter is to explore this aspect of the new discourse of health.

To do so, we discuss gender and health in three ways. First, we consider how the problem of women's health has been defined in the past, to draw attention to some differences with today. Second, we detail some of the main features of the contemporary problem of men's health. Finally, we use the case study of campaigns about cancer screening, to illustrate the nature of, and problems with, this aspect of the new discourse of health.

The problem of 'women's health'

In contemporary society, attitudes and behaviours – in particular those considered to be associated with 'masculinity' – have come to be defined as 'unhealthy'. The construction of health concerns in terms of gender is a fairly recent phenomenon. The gendering of health is a development inextricably linked to the second-wave feminist movement, a movement that made the relationship between women, medicine and society a matter of significant public debate and contest. The development of the term 'medicalisation' – defined sociologically as the process through which experiences come to be understood in medical terms – is strongly associated with this historical development.[4] Employed to explore a range of experiences it is aspects of women's lives that have been particularly subject to analysis through use of this term by feminists.[5]

Feminist literature from the 1970s and 1980s 'emphasized the breadth of the medicalization of women's lives', notes Conrad.[6] Where women's lives were described and analysed as subject to medicalisation, at this time it tended to be the *problematic* effects of this process that were emphasised. As Reismann put it in her oft-quoted contribution on the subject, women were viewed as the 'main targets' of the medicalisation processes, indicating that the definition of women's experiences in terms of illness was considered to be negative. 'A plethora of female conditions has come to be … reconceptualized as illnesses' she wrote, citing as examples sexual dysfunctions, pregnancy care, fertility, menopause, ageing, teenage pregnancy and wife battering, premenstrual syndrome, and weight gain.[7]

Why did feminists respond to illness definitions in this way? One objection to medicalised accounts of womens experiences is that they *naturalise* demeaning and degrading ideas about women, a point made in one of the founding feminist statements about the problem of medicalisation, by Barbara Ehrenreich and Diedre English:

> The medical system is strategic for women's liberation … It holds the promise of freedom from hundreds of unspoken fears and complaints that have handicapped women throughout history … But the medical system is also strategic to women's oppression. Medical science has been one of the most powerful sources of sexist ideology in our culture. Justifications for sexual discrimination – in education, in jobs, in public life – must ultimately rest on one thing that differentiates women from men: their bodies. Theories of male superiority ultimately rest on biology.[8]

Medicalised explanations for women's experience 'reduce women to their biology' it was argued, by explaining sex differences in society with reference to reproductive organs and hormones. In turn explanations of this sort continually draw attention to the idea that women are ill. 'Medicine's prime contribution to sexist ideology has been to describe women as sick, and as potentially sickening to men', stated Ehrenreich and English. Women throughout history have been considered 'the weaker sex' and excluded from major areas of social life on these grounds, they claimed, an outcome they described through discussion of nineteenth-century '"sick" women of the upper classes', made hypochondriac and hysterical through a life of enforced leisure, and the 'sickening women of the working classes', deemed a threat to social order in general and to children in particular. Medicine in this framework was viewed as one, very powerful, aspect, of an overall 'sexist ideology', and concepts such as 'hysteria' and 'pre-menstrual syndrome' were contested and objected to for this reason.

Another important theme in the discussion of medicalisation emphasised that medical interventions can *disempower* women. While medicine promised 'liberation and freedom' through, for example, enabling women to effectively regulate their fertility by using contraception and abortion, women's experience in practice was very different, argued some. An outlook of protest regarding medical interventions emerged as a result, described in 1976 by the feminist sociologist Ann Oakley:

> These protests cover such topics as the undue use of surgical abortion techniques ... the overuse of radical as opposed to constructive surgery for breast and reproductive tract diseases ... and perhaps, most central of all, the modern, male-controlled, hospitalised and increasingly technological pattern of childbirth management.[9]

Medical care for women, it was claimed, failed to reflect women's needs and interests, a problem most clearly apparent when women experienced childbirth. Through the modern profession of obstetrics and the development of hospital-based childbirth, feminist critics claimed pregnant women had come to be construed as patients, with healthy women treated as if they were sick, and women's pregnancy and childbirth experiences consequently controlled by the medical profession.[10] Women's own control over their bodies and reproductive experience was for this reason diminished and childbirth emerged as probably the key area for criticism of medicalisation.

Some saw alternative health care as a solution, and they set up their own health care provision. The best-known project of this kind was the Boston Women's Health Collective which advocated self-help for women, rather than reliance on doctors, and whose manual *Our Bodies Ourselves* first published in 1972 rapidly made an international impact. In the Preface it states, of the women who set up the Collective:

> We had all experienced similar feelings of frustration and anger towards specific doctors and the medical maze in general, and initially we wanted to do something about those doctors who were condescending, paternalistic, judgemental, and non-informative ... [over time] we realised we really were capable of collecting, understanding and evaluating medical information.[11]

Exemplifying the spirit of defiance informing this approach was the Chicago-based underground abortion service 'Jane'. Set up when abortion was still illegal in the USA by women who believed abortion to be a basic precondition of women's equality,

'Jane' was staffed by a group of women who, first under the guidance of a doctor, trained themselves to perform abortion, and eventually carried out around 11,000 safe and successful abortion procedures during the early 1970s.[12] Such initiatives were more prominent in the USA and Australia, although there were attempts by British feminists to provide alternatives to mainstream medicine.[13]

There has been much debate about these feminist criticisms of modern medicine. One area of dispute concerns historical accuracy. Some feminist representations of modern medical care have implied there was once a 'golden age' of woman-centred 'natural childbirth', but little evidence has been presented to substantiate this claim. Such claims also run counter to evidence of a somewhat barbaric experience that led *women* to *demand* precisely the interventions subsequently represented as part of the unwelcome medicalisation of childbirth – for example drug-based pain relief.[14] Indeed, 'the movement for "natural" childbirth only arose when medical advances had freed women from these fears [of the pain of childbirth]', argued Strong.[15] In turn it has been suggested that there is no good reason to assume that female-dominated midwifery is 'good' for women, and high-tech reproductive medicine 'bad'.[16]

The 1980s and 1990s saw the emergence of arguments that approached the problem of 'women's health' in a way that departed from that of the 1970s.[17] Some have revised the original feminist formulation of the problem of medicalisation, in order to emphasise the possibility of women benefiting from and taking advantage of modern medicine. Attention has been drawn to the diversity of women's experiences of healthcare; women can and do benefit from mainstream medical treatment and are not passive recipients of it, it has been argued.[18] 'It is now difficult to identify a single feminist critique of medicine. Instead a variety of feminist approaches to health and health care have emerged', concludes Doyal of these developments.[19]

In relation to the main subject area of this chapter – the rise of concern about men's health – a third difference between feminist definitions of the problem of women's health in the 1970s, and more recent claims about this social problem are important. The former, as we have emphasised, articulated suspicion about female acquiescence to medical authority and intervention, and some on this basis made bold attempts to provide alternatives to mainstream medicine. In contrast, the problem of women's health is today often defined quite differently. It tends to be the *absence* of official, medical intervention that is bemoaned, and the need for *more* professional help is advocated. As we will go on to argue, it is this sort of approach, rather than that apparent in earlier decades, that has crossed the gender divide, and underpins the approach of those who argue that more needs to be done about men's health.

Take, for example, post-natal depression (PND). This psychiatric category was rejected at one time by many feminists for medicalising maternal experience and misrepresenting its nature.[20] More recently, in contrast, the category PND has come to be widely embraced as a useful term to describe how new mothers feel. A burgeoning body of literature emerged through the 1990s, including titles such as *Surviving Post-natal Depression* and *The New Mother Syndrome: Coping with Postpartum Stress and Depression*. The over-riding message of these books is that women have been left by doctors to 'suffer in silence', and it is vital that society, and in particular the medical profession, does more to recognise and diagnose PND and encourage women to seek medical help. The project of the authors of such books is to *generalise* the incidence of PND, so that most mothers come to be defined as victims of it. Thus the writer Kate Figes, in her widely read advice book for new mothers, argues, 'It [PND] is a sliding scale, starting with the "baby blues" affecting 80 per cent of women, and ending with puerperal psychosis ... The vast majority of women sit somewhere on this scale'.[21] Interestingly, some feminists share this approach. American feminist Naomi Wolf for example claims that 400,000 American mothers each year are affected by depression after they have a baby, and she highlights what she sees as 'medical complacency in the face of women's suffering', because routine screening for post-natal depression is not normally provided in the USA by doctors.[22]

Post-natal Depression has thus come to be represented as common in one form or another to all mothers, and in turn most mothers are deemed in need of medical diagnosis and treatment. The demand is for *more diagnosis not less*, and this demand is not restricted to PND. Many illness categories, including pre-menstrual syndrome and post-traumatic stress disorder are discussed as 'hidden epidemics' that need to be more widely diagnosed in women by doctors. In recent years new categories of illness including Battered Women's Syndrome, Rape Trauma Syndrome and Childbirth Trauma Syndrome have been 'named' and their medical diagnosis promoted by some.[23] Some campaigners also argue that women need more screening of the cervix and breast, and more advice and guidance from doctors about issues including weight gain, weight loss, exercise, and pregnancy.

If in the past the problem of women's health was shaped by a feminist approach that comprised in part at least the defiant rejection of official illness categories, this suggests that other definitions of health and illness are now ascendant. The forthright message that women should resist the unwelcome foisting of medical labels and treatments upon them has waned, and the stronger tendency has been towards the emergence of the contrasting notion that *too little* is done by society to allow women to recognise their health problems. One implication of this redefinition of the problem of women's health is a shift in emphasis regarding the value of the 'feminine' and the 'masculine'.

Agnes Miles has explained this point, with reference to the work of the feminist critic of psychiatry, Philys Chesler. Chesler explained, in her account of why objections should be raised regarding 'the feminine' in the context of health and medicine, that 'women are socialized and pressed into accepting the feminine role, which is compatible with the position of a submissive and dependent help-seeker'. The role of help-seeker is a 'dependent and submissive one', she thus explained. For Chesler, in other words, 'help-seeking' was an outlook bound up with 'feminine' attitudes of passivity and submission which women were socialised to adopt.[24]

This point was made by Chesler as part of an account of why women were more likely to feel ill and visit doctors than men, and her emphasis was on the connection between 'help-seeking' and a damaging and negative socio-cultural context for women. The now widespread advocacy of the *positive* value of help-seeking draws attention to the extent to which a new validation of 'the feminine' has emerged. As we now detail, it is this development above all that is made manifest by campaigns about 'men's health'.

Men's health and the problem of 'masculinity'

Within twenty years the feminist campaign to seize control over women's health from the medical profession has given way to a state-sponsored, doctor-led system of vaginal examination and cervical surveillance. It is doubly ironic that within the same period, male resistance to medical regulation was replaced by the demand, under the banner of 'men's health', for invasive screening tests analogous to cervical smears.[25]

The problem of 'men's health' has, as Fitzpatrick acerbically indicates, rapidly gained visibility and recognition. Twenty years ago, there was no such problem. Men of course more or less willingly visited doctors when confronted by symptoms of ill health. But there were few active efforts to encourage men to become concerned about their health. Since the early 1990s, however, activities and initiatives that seek to bring the problem of men's health to public attention, and which in particular aim to change the attitudes and behaviour of men themselves, have become a ubiquitous feature of social life.

The most obvious example of this new preoccupation is the emergence of a specialist popular literature for men about their health. Traditionally marketed for women, men's health magazines first appeared on the British market just over a decade ago.[26] It was at about the same time that campaign groups were established to 'raise awareness' of 'men's health needs'. The best-known and most influential such British group, Men's Health Forum was founded in 1994.[27] Little more than ten years later, such initiatives are numerous and very visible. Male students at the University of Kent are welcomed to their campus with posters asking them whether they have recently examined their testicles, and encouraging them to visit the doctor if they have not. Awareness campaigns of this type are now commonplace. A wide range of projects seek to promote the need for male awareness of conditions ranging from prostate, testicular and breast cancer, to anorexia and bulimia, post-natal depression and heart disease. What are the features of this new health concern? Four themes can be identified.

The bifurcation of health concerns

One of the most notable aspects of men's health concerns is the way advocates of their recognition often self-consciously challenge sex-based distinctions associated with health campaigns in the past. Men are the 'forgotten victims' of post-natal depression, argues the author of one book on the subject, since 'becoming a father can have a huge impact on a man and yet all the attention seems to be focused on the woman'.[28] Male cancers such as prostate and testicular cancer are promoted as important health problems that should be taken as seriously as breast cancer, and breast cancer itself is now defined as an under-recognised men's health problem. The menopause has also crossed the sex divide, with some claiming it affects men in middle age as well as women.

The health of young men and boys has become a particular focus for claims of this kind. Anorexia and deliberate self-harm in the past considered psychological problems associated most often with young women, are thus represented as disorders that affect more and more young men. The problem of 'poor sexual health' is also now widely considered to be a male as much as female problem with claims made that boys in particular need to be targeted in programmes that aim to improve sexual health, and combat teenage pregnancy. The process of 'medicalization' – the definition of social experience in medical terms – has, as was noted earlier, been strongly associated in sociological literature with the experiences of women. As Rosenfeld and Faircloth detail however, this sort of contemporary experience suggests there is now a strong tendency for men's lives to also be increasingly medicalized.[29]

A common diagnosis for a range of conditions

A second feature of the problem of men's health is that a wide range of different diseases and complaints, which have very little in common in a medical sense, are united by one common diagnosis. Taking as their central trope the idea of 'traditional masculinity', advocates of greater recognition for the problem of men's health blame ill health in men – in whichever form it might appear – on a particular set of attitudes and sensibilities. Regardless of which men's health problem is at issue, the ultimate cause of the problem – 'masculinity' – is always the same.

Thus argued one early advocate of the need for more to done about men's health, 'The road to improvement in men's health lies in puncturing typical myths of masculinity such as that it's good to be daring, unemotional and in control'.[30] In this framework, it is men's attitudes, their alleged 'daring' and 'unemotional' outlook that constitutes the barrier to health, regardless of which medical problem is at issue.

Social psychologists Lee and Owens also centre their analysis on 'hegemonic masculinity', defined as 'toughness, unemotionality, physical competence, competitiveness and aggression'.[31] Illness-inducing behaviours associated with 'hegemonic masculinity', they claim, include 'relative reluctance to seek help for medical and psychological problems', 'avoidance of the expression of emotion', and 'a high level of involvement in risky behaviours, which include both the socially sanctioned risks involved in dangerous sports and the more deviant masculine-type risks such as crime and violent behaviour'. Similarly, according to one health website, it is 'male stereotypes' that damage men's health, centrally the 'macho' stereotype that centres on 'an inability to admit vulnerability'.[32] In this framework, ill health of all types is thus commonly caused by a particular form of identity, that which is 'masculine', meaning it is only when men adopt a different set of attitudes, crucially those that involve a 'feminine' acceptance of vulnerability, and embrace the need to seek help, that health can be attained.

'Men's health' as a socio-cultural problem

The speed at which men's lives and experiences have been medicalised points to the conclusion that developments in science and medicine cannot be solely responsible for this development. It would be difficult for even the most energetic and enthusiastic 'medical imperialists' to generate the degree of interest in men's behaviour and attitudes that now exists, suggesting there has been a *broader socio-cultural shift*. Certain perceptions of what is positive or negative about attitudes and behaviour have come to be socially and culturally validated, and these perceptions have been imported into debates about health. The idea that 'masculinity' is a plastic set of attitudes and behaviours that can and should be modified is associated originally with the fields of sociology and social psychology.[33] Through a process of cultural transmission, it seems such theories about men and their (allegedly problematic) behaviour have come to influence much wider arenas, including the medical.

A problem definition that influences the medical world

The way that men think about themselves can be quite unhelpful ... Most men don't like to admit that they feel fragile or vulnerable, and so are less likely to talk about their feelings with their friends, loved ones or their doctors. This may be the reason that they often don't ask for help when they become depressed.

Concerns about 'masculine', 'unhealthy' behaviour and attitudes, if non-medical in origin, have come to be strongly endorsed by the medical world. The degree to which 'masculine' values and attitudes have been stigmatised (and 'feminine' ones validated) is indicated by the extent to which the claim that men need to be encouraged to be less 'tough', 'invulnerable' and 'in control', and more 'open', 'soft', and prepared to 'seek help' informs health-related institutions, and the medical profession itself. Despite the dubious efficacy of almost all interventions for men justified on such grounds many medical bodies endorse the idea that there is need to address men's health in this way.[35]

The Royal College of Nursing, the British Medical Association and the Royal College of Psychiatrists all have initiatives that aim to encourage men to seek help and which aim to counter the allegedly detrimental effects of 'masculinity' for health. In 2005 a range of international medical societies came together in Vienna for a 'World Congress on Men's Health and Gender'. '[M]en's health is much more than just about diseases that affect men', argues the doctor who organised the conference. 'It is also about the consequences of male attitudes to health in general', he claimed.[36] Official health promotion programmes in Britain explicitly target men on just this basis[37] and key organisations also promote the need to change 'men's attitudes'.

In summary, the growing visibility of the problem of men's health implies cultural stigmatisation of particular attitudes, for example resilience, and the validation of others, for example risk aversion and help-seeking. This in turn implies a significant increase in the medicalisation of men's lives, as men are encouraged to seek help, if possible in advance of any symptom of ill health. It is for this reason that, on the one hand, the alleged reluctance on the part of men to go to the doctor is bemoaned, and on the other, regardless of their dubious efficacy, programmes that seek to encourage more men (and women) to take up preventative health measures are championed.

It is perhaps the advocacy of screening programmes for cancer that illustrates most clearly the central aspects of the changing definitions of gender and health discussed so far. It is to this case study of the 'feminization' of health that we now turn.

Cancer and cancer screening

It is hardly possible to take up one's residence in the kingdom of the ill unprejudiced by the lurid metaphors with which it has been landscaped.[38]

In the 1970s Susan Sontag wrote, in her book *Illness as Metaphor*, about the social stigma of the cancer sufferer. She described the metaphors and mythology surrounding cancer, and the way this mystification made it harder for cancer sufferers to come to terms with their illness as an illness.

In recent years, cancer has been demystified, both in medical terms, and also in terms of public discourse. The gradual introduction of more effective treatments, in some cases cures, alongside development of a more interventionist model of palliative care have meant that in western societies, the burden of physical suffering caused by cancer is considerably reduced. The theories Sontag describes about the psychological basis of cancer, from Galen's description of 'melancholy women' in the second century to the 1970s 'cancer personality' (depressive, repressed, with poor relationship skills) have been overturned, and now seem unscientific and indeed cruel, as we have learned more about the genetic and environmental causes of the disease. Sontag describes a French oncologist who told her that less than a tenth of his patients knew they had cancer. Only 30 years later, this level of denial seems unimaginable.

It would be wrong to draw the conclusion that mythology about cancer has disappeared, however. Some of today's beliefs about cancer are summed up in the opening paragraphs of the Haynes *Men's Cancer Manual* from 2004: 'although about one man in three will develop a cancer at some time in his life, the most common forms are almost entirely preventable or treatable through early diagnosis'. In other words, it is suggested that if we behave responsibly, by reporting suspicious symptoms to our doctors, and following the type of lifestyle advice contained in the Haynes manual, we may avoid cancer altogether or certainly drastically improve our chances of survival. The message of this campaign is that 'awareness saves lives'. As we shall see however this simple, apparently commonsensical message is unfortunately not borne out by the evidence. The real impact of 'awareness campaigns' is not less cancer, but ironically a higher incidence of cancer, along with a new consciousness of the possibility of becoming sick, and further legitimation of help-seeking behaviour.

Breast cancer

Cancer campaigns have gained enormous popularity and publicity in the UK and USA. Take the example of breast cancer. Three-quarters of a million women were expected to take part in the 'Race for Life' in 2006, a three-mile run organised by the UK charity Cancer Research. Over a million take part in the annual 'Race for the Cure', the US equivalent. Barbara Ehrenreich wrote about this popular movement after she was diagnosed with breast cancer herself:

> Culture is too weak a word to describe all this. What has grown up in just the last fifteen years more nearly represents a cult – or given that it numbers more than two million women, their families and their friends – perhaps we should say a full-fledged religion.[39]

The roots of this 'religion' arguably lie in aspects of the feminist movement of which Ehrenreich herself was a part. In the 1970s, the impact of the women's movement in relation to breast cancer was two-fold. First, women were encouraged to be more open about their bodies and diseases. Various American celebrities of the time 'went public' about their breast cancer and treatment, notably First Lady Betty Ford, newsreader Betty Rollin, tycoon's wife Happy Rockefeller and former child actor

Shirley Temple Black. Black justified her decision to speak out in early 1972 as one made 'for all my sisters who have lost a breast, for all my sisters who fear they may'. Second, the women's movement was an important part of the drive towards more conservative, less disfiguring treatment for breast cancer, which formed part of its criticism of medical control of women. In the words of Black again: 'The doctor can make the incision, I'll make the decision'.[40]

This challenge to medical paternalism had a real impact. Combined with new medical advances and understanding about the way cancer spread, it brought improved treatment to sufferers. The contribution of feminism to the eventual death-knoll of the radical Halsted mastectomy (involving removal of the breast, chest muscles and axillary lymph-nodes) practised since the 1890s has been described this way:

> Transforming the prevailing mind-set would take more, much more, than data, statistics and refereed articles in scientific journals. American surgeons did not come around for years, not until the sexual revolution and modern feminism altered the cultural and political landscape, changing forever American attitudes about power, eroticism and physical beauty.[41]

What is different about today's breast cancer campaigners? The emphasis on the 'survivor' speaking out is still with us. Indeed, for breast cancer sufferers in the public eye, it now seems almost obligatory. When pop singer Kylie Minogue was diagnosed in 2005, the details of her subsequent surgery made headline news. There was never any question that Minogue had a choice in the public discussion of her medical problems, as her surgeon gave daily press briefings on the hospital steps. She was congratulated by the press as she issued statements denying that she was using alternative therapies, conscious of the influence attached to her celebrity.

But Minogue's case shows how the aim of 'speaking out' has changed. Her situation was used not to challenge medical control, but as an opportunity to educate others about 'breast cancer awareness'. Television news interviewers approached random young women in the street, asking them whether they examined their own breasts for signs of cancer and sought medical advice. Rates of young women requesting mammograms soared in Minogue's native Australia. The role of the celebrity survivor today is thus not to help women find an independent way to respond to an illness, but rather to encourage as many people as possible to be 'aware' and take the advice of cancer campaigners and charities, and seek help from doctors in the form of cancer screening.

Rather than struggling to free women from unnecessary tests and over-treatment by a conservative medical profession, today's campaigners seem relatively unquestioning about the need for as many tests and as much treatment as possible. The charity Breast Cancer Care has thus recently organised a specific campaign to raise breast awareness among black and ethnic minority (BME) women in Britain, and publicised the following comment:

> 43 per cent of BME women said they never look at or feel their breasts. 45 per cent of BME women of screening age (50 to 70 years) had never attended the NHS breast cancer screening programme. Breast Cancer Care is committed to ensuring that everyone in the UK has access to high quality breast awareness and breast cancer information. We believe this is an essential part of strategies to increase early detection.[42]

The justification for raising awareness here is increasing early detection, as women will be encouraged to examine their breasts and go for screening. Although this is not spelled out, the implicit presumption is that this will also improve women's chances of surviving breast cancer, yet problems can be identified with this idea.

Perhaps surprisingly this idea is not borne out by the medical evidence. Take breast self-examination, until recently a central facet of awareness campaigns. For many years, women were encouraged to use a technique similar to that used by medical practitioners to examine their own breasts, looking for suspicious signs of cancer. Several trials have discovered that not only is this not beneficial, it is overall a harmful exercise.[43] Groups of women who were taught how to examine their breasts were compared with those who were not, and the results showed no difference in mortality between the two groups, but an increase in potentially harmful benign breast biopsies in the group examining themselves.

The benefits of mammography, used widely to screen for breast cancer, are also contested in medical circles. A review in October 2006, by the highly respected Cochrane group, suggested that

> for every 2000 women invited for screening throughout 10 years, one will have her life prolonged. In addition, 10 healthy women, who would not have been diagnosed if there had not been screening, will be diagnosed as breast cancer patients and will be treated unnecessarily. It is thus not clear whether screening does more good than harm. Women invited to screening should be fully informed of both benefits and harms.[44]

This caution regarding efficacy is rarely expressed by breast cancer charities, and it is particularly the failure to provide clear information and advice to women which incenses critics of breast cancer screening. Informed choice, one of the buzzwords of modern medicine, is often overlooked in promotion of mammography according to the UK breast surgeon Professor Michael Baum:

> Tensions exist between the demands of the screening industry's 'pursuit of good uptake' and properly promoting informed choice of patients ... Most women who are screened have neither suffered nor been educated about the reality of the uncertainties, harms, and limitations of screening or the consequences of finding pathology of borderline importance.[45]

One Australian study reviewed 58 leaflets given to women to explain mammography.[46] The researchers found that the leaflets were much more likely to quote the statistics for lifetime risk of breast cancer (1 in 10 by the age of 85) rather than the lifetime risk of dying from breast cancer (about 3 in 100). Benefits of mammography were explained in terms of relative risk reduction, with estimates from 30–50 per cent improved survival (estimates which it would be difficult to support from medical literature). No leaflets at all cited the more prosaic 'number needed to treat' format, as used by the Cochrane review mentioned earlier.

This disregard for medical evidence seems to indicate that the goal of awareness has become an end in itself. Indeed, in the words of Breast Cancer Care's literature, 'The campaign seeks to emphasise that anyone can be affected by breast cancer, whatever their background, and everyone should be breast aware'.[47] There is a moral imperative here, in the demand that all of us should live life with an awareness of mortality and human susceptibility to disease, regardless of the relatively low risks the disease poses for a particular individual. In this regard, it has been argued that some contemporary cancer campaigns misrepresent the medical evidence. The imperative to 'be aware' also creates new difficulties.

The effects of 'awareness' are perhaps shown most clearly in the display of the pink ribbon. A tenet of breast cancer campaigning is that women are encouraged to identify their support and awareness publicly, a trend epitomised by ribbon wearing. Sarah Moore investigated this fashion in her research. She interviewed a group of women about why they wore pink ribbons, and her findings make for interesting reading.

'Because it's your worst fear, to have breast cancer', stated one woman, who Moore describes as 'often reticent ... [she] frequently spoke in a whispered tone'. She describes another interviewee whose mother had recently recovered from breast cancer. She explained wearing a pink ribbon as a means of reminding herself of the risks associated with the disease:

Every time I put my coat on [and see the ribbon] I'm remembering that this thing's going to be in my mum's body for the rest of her life. And it could happen to me. You've got to be aware that it could happen to you ... I obviously don't sit there everyday thinking, "Oh, I could have breast cancer. I could get breast cancer". It's just one of those subconscious things that rushes across your mind in a matter of seconds when you put your coat on and see the ribbon.[48]

Most of her interviewees described ribbon wearing in terms of worries or fears about the disease. The consciousness or awareness of illness so sought after by campaigners is thus revealed not as a positive, helpful force in their lives but as a 'constant, niggling sense of worry about this illness'. What was also interesting about Moore's interviewees is that they were mostly young women. Given that only around 2000 UK women under 40 are diagnosed with breast cancer each year, the impact of such worries seems to fall unfairly on their shoulders.

Testicular and prostate cancers

The successes of the contemporary breast cancer lobby have inspired others to follow directly in their footsteps. Charities funding research into cancers affecting men, particularly prostate cancer and testicular cancer, have followed the 'awareness-raising' model in their own campaigning. In place of pink ribbons and girly T-shirts, are beer-mats and 'Prostate cancer tool-kits™'.

Even more than is apparent in breast cancer campaigning, 'raising awareness' is promoted as a primary goal for men's cancer campaigns. The assumption underlying the men's health movement, that 'masculinity' makes men ignorant about their own bodies and health, and too reluctant to seek help, leads to the claim they need to be persuaded to do so by whatever means necessary.

Colin Osborne, who set up the Orchid Appeal, a charity raising awareness of testicular cancer, thus described himself prior to diagnosis as 'not one to go to the doctor's ... I have to be at death's door before I stop what I'm doing'.[49] It might be said that this happy-go-lucky attitude is quite reasonable for a young man in the prime of life. Testicular cancer is extremely rare, and has better cure rates than any other cancer (95%, even for those with advanced disease). There is no need for young men to worry about this disease. Yet Osborne has drawn the opposite conclusion, despite evidence to the contrary. He represents this 'masculine' disregard for ill health as dangerous and unwise and encourages other men to change their outlook on life if they are to avoid suffering from the problems he has faced.

In 2003 the Prostate Research Campaign ran a campaign called *Ignorance Isn't Bliss*. This campaign sought to encourage women to 'persuade your man to talk to his doctor about his prostate health'. Leaflets advised women to 'leave medical information leaflets lying around where he is likely to find them – i.e., the bathroom, near the remote control or on the car seat'. 'Feminine' acceptance of the need to seek help is thus envisaged as the means to change the way men behave. As one general practitioner put it, recognising the moral imperative regarding behaviour in such campaigns, 'The unfortunate conclusion I fear from reading the leaflet is that good men get PSA tests done, and good women make sure of it'.[50]

Prostate cancer is unusual in that it more often than not causes no problematic symptoms. Post-mortem studies have shown that around 40 per cent of men who die aged over 70 have prostate cancer.[51] In the past, most of them would have been blissfully unaware of this fact. The introduction of the prostate-specific antigen (PSA) blood test in the late 1980s has caused an enormous increase in the number of men diagnosed with prostate cancer (almost doubling in the USA). More than any other cancer, however, screening and early treatment for prostate cancer are highly controversial. In the UK, there is no organised screening for prostate cancer precisely because of the lack of evidence that screening is helpful, and evidence of its potential harmfulness.

Problematically, PSA testing does not differentiate between aggressive and potentially fatal cancers, and those that might have had a benign course, never troubling their host. Many more of these formerly hidden and harmless prostate cancers are now being picked up. One critic has accurately described this as 'the eradication of a disease: how we cured symptomless prostate cancer'. Formerly symptomless prostate cancer now has a new symptom, 'a disabling state of anxiety resulting from (men's) knowledge of their PSA level'.[52]

Just as we have seen in the case of breast cancer, evidence of the harms of 'awareness' and the advocacy of 'help seeking' does not, however, deter the campaigners. Medical intervention in the most personal aspects of men's lives is welcomed. For example, the Prostate Cancer Charity sells the 'Peeball™', a biodegradable ball that men can destroy by urinating on. This is marketed as a fun game to be played in pub toilets with friends, but of course it contains a serious message. The charity's website warns, 'It is not a diagnostic tool to test for prostate cancer. However difficulty passing urine whilst playing the game may indicate a prostate or urinary problem'.[53] This is reminiscent of Barbara Ehrenreich's description of the 'infantilizing trope' of merchandise such as teddy bears and crayons sold in aid of breast cancer charities.

In summary, the new discourse of health, as we described earlier, makes modifying the 'internal life' of individuals central to the pursuit of health. Campaigns for cancer awareness strongly exemplify and express this approach to 'health'. Yet such campaigns can have a highly negative effect at the level of the individual, in terms of raised anxiety levels and unnecessary medical interventions. One critic has contrasted such campaigns with the ideals of the women's movement in the 1970s, which attempted to resist the medical profession's intervention into the intimacies of everyday life:

Just as the smear test exposes women not merely to the medical gaze but to vaginal penetration, so the palpation of the prostate involves digital penetration of the male rectum. The slippery finger may be less impressive than the metal speculum, but it is no less significant an instrument of domination.[54]

On a broader social level, we have arguably moved from the state of denial described by Sontag to a position where we are all encouraged to see ourselves as 'cancer victims in-waiting'.

Conclusion

The problem of women's health came to prominence because of second-wave feminism in the 1970s. Discussion of the relationship between gender and health has a longer history however. The feminist novelist Virginia Woolf wrote in 1929:

In a hundred years ... women will have ceased to be the protected sex ... All assumptions founded on the facts observed when women were the protected sex will have disappeared – as, for example, that women and clergymen and gardeners live longer than other people. Remove that protection, expose them to the same exertions and activities, make them soldiers and sailors and engine drivers and dock-labourers, and will not women die off so much younger, so much quicker.[55]

What mattered to Woolf was for women to be equal to men, and no longer the 'protected sex'. The most rewarding objective of life for women as well as men was, as far as she was concerned 'exertion and activity'. Almost 100 years later women are no longer the 'protected sex' they once were, but aspects of the new-found equality between women and men appear very different to that Woolf imagined, when she thought of the equal society of the future.

In the age of the new discourse of health a code of conduct has developed to shape the behaviour of both sexes, which is a far cry from Woolf's vision of what might lie ahead. Epitomised by advice given about men's health, it is one that upholds the 'virtues of the feminine'. Admission of vulnerability, risk awareness, and help-seeking behaviour are championed as desirable attributes for both men and women. It might be argued that, in Woolf's terms, both men and women are in this way encouraged to adopt the identity of 'the protected sex'. What should we make of this outcome? Do we live in a better society because of this?

This chapter has argued that the cultural dominance of the new discourse of health, with its mantra 'prevention is better than cure', should be assessed very critically. The preventative approach now advocated so widely may appear to be 'common sense'. Yet closer examination suggests it may have the effect of encouraging *illness identities*. Our discussion has suggested that control of health 'from the inside' through 'awareness raising' involves encouraging people to adopt the identity of the help seeker, in contrast to that of the 'invulnerable' person, who assumes they are well most of the time. Could an unintended consequence of this strategy for improving the health of the nation be to make more people than ever worried about being ill? Could it even be that people come to consider themselves ill in this context?

Discussion topics

- Why is 'masculinity' considered a cause of ill health?
- Why might it be argued that preventative health programmes seek to modify identity, or 'control health from within'?
- How and why has cancer changed in the public imagination? What are the possible effects of increased cancer awareness among men?

Further reading

Lee, E. (2003) *Abortion, Motherhood and Mental Health: Medicalizing Reproduction in the United States and Great Britain.* New York: Transaction.

This book uses the examples of Post-abortion Syndrome and Post-natal Depression to explore how women's experiences of pregnancy have been pathologised. It is also a useful read for those interested in how sociologists go about exploring the construction of social problems.

Olson, J. (2002) *Bathsheba's Breast: Women, Cancer and History.* Baltimore, MD: Johns Hopkins University Press.

American historian James Olson explores the history of breast cancer through the ages, from the sufferings of Persian queen Atossa in 538 B.C. to Jerri Nielsen's confrontation with cancer at the South Pole in A.D. 1999. He describes how developments in medical understanding and treatment have interacted with cultural factors, in particular the rise of feminism and patient activism.

Rosenfeld, D. and Faircloth, C.A. (eds), (2006) *Medicalized Masculinities.* Philadelphia, PA: Temple University Press.

In this edited collection, contributors discuss a range of ways in which men's lives have been medicalised; chapters discuss issues including balding, viagra, boys and ADHD and war veterans and PTSD. The Introduction provides a very useful overview of how sociology might theorise the medicalisation of masculinity.

References

1   Nettleton, S. (2006) *The Sociology of Health and Illness.* Cambridge: Polity.
2   Nettleton, S. (2006) ibid., p. 244, emphasis in the original.
3   Kimmel, M.S. (1995) Series editor's introduction. In D. Sabo and D.F. Gordon (eds), *Men's Health and Illness.* London: Sage, pp. vii–viii.
4   Rosenfeld, D. (2006) Medicalized masculinities: the missing link? In D. Rosenfeld and C.A. Faircloth (eds), *Medicalized Masculinities.* Philadelphia, PA: Temple University Press.
5   See for example, Zola, I.K. (1972/1978) Medicine as an institution of social control. In J. Ehrenreich and B. Eherenreich (eds), *The Cultural Crisis of Modern Medicine.*

New York and London: Monthly Review Press, pp. 80–100; Conrad, P. (1992) Medicalization and social control. *Annual Review of Sociology*, 18: 209–32; and Gabe, J., Bury, M. and Elston, M.A. (2004) *Key Concepts in Medical Sociology* ('Medicalization'). London: Sage. Also Furedi F., this volume.

6 Conrad, P. (1992) ibid., p. 222.

7 Riessman, C.K. (1983) Women and medicalization: a new perspective. *Social Policy*, Summer: 3–17.

8 Ehrenreich, B. and English, D. (1973) *Complaints and Disorders: The Sexual Politics of Sickness*. New York: The Feminist Press.

9 Oakley, A. (1976) Wisewoman and medicine man: changes in the management of childbirth. In A. Oakley and J. Mitchell (eds), *The Rights and Wrongs of Women*. Harmondsworth: Penguin, pp. 52–3.

10 Graham, H. and Oakley, A. (1981) Competing ideologies of reproduction: medical and maternal perspectives in pregnancy. In H. Roberts (ed.), *Women, Health and Reproduction*. London: Routledge and Kegan Paul.

11 Boston Women's Health Book Collective (1995) Our bodies ourselves. In M. Schneir (ed.), *The Vintage Book of Feminism*. London: Vintage, p. 353.

12 Gordon, L. (1990) *Woman's Body, Woman's Right*. New York: Penguin.

13 Doyal, L. (1994) Changing medicine? Gender and the politics of healthcare. In J. Gabe, D. Kelleher and G. Williams (eds), *Challenging Medicine*. London: Routledge.

14 Shorter, E. (1997) *Women's Bodies*. New Brunswick, NJ: Transaction.

15 Strong, P.M. (1979) Sociological imperialism and the profession of medicine. *Social Science and Medicine*, 13A: 199–215.

16 Annandale, E.C. and Clark, J. (1996) What is gender? Feminist theory and the sociology of human reproduction. *Sociology of Health and Illness*, 18(1): 17–44.

17 White, K. (2002) *An Introduction to the Sociology of Health and Illness*. London: Sage Publications.

18 See Purdy, L. (2001) Medicalization, medical necessity, and feminist medicine. *Bioethics*, 15(3): 248–61 and Gabe, J., Bury, M. and Elston, M.A. (2004) *Key Concepts in Medical Sociology* ('Reproduction'). London: Sage.

19 Doyal, L. (1994) ibid., p. 142.

20 Miles, A. (1991) *Women, Health and Medicine*. Milton Keynes: Open University Press.

21 Figes, K. (1998) *Life After Birth*. London: Penguin, p. 40.

22 Wolf, N. (2001) *Misconceptions, Truth, Lies and the Unexpected on the Journey to Motherhood*. London: Chatto and Windus, p. 184.

23 For discussion of this subject, see Downs, D. (1996) *More Than Victims, Battered Women, the Syndrome Society and the Law*. Chicago: The University of Chicago Press; Figert, A.E. (1996) *Women and the Ownership of PMS: The Structuring of a Psychiatric Disorder*. New York: Aldine de Gruyter; Lee, E. (2003) *Abortion, motherhood and mental health: medicalizing reproduction in the United States and Great Britain*. New York: Transaction; Raitt, F.E. and Zeedyk, S. (2000) *The Implicit Relation of Psychology and Law, Women and Syndrome Evidence*. London: Routledge; and Westervelt, S.D. (1998) *Shifting the Blame: How Victimization Became a Criminal Defense*. New Brunswick, NJ: Rutgers University Press.

24 Miles, A. (1991) ibid., p. 65.

25 Fitzpatrick, M. (2001) *The Tyranny of Health*. London: Routledge.

26 Tredre, R. (1992) American magazine's target Britain's new men. *The Independent*.

27 Baker, P. (1994) Focus on men: sorry for the horrors, doctor. The Men's Health Network. The *Independent*, p. 20; Men's Health Forum. 'About Us', http//www.menshelathforum.org.uk

28 Curham, S. (2000) *Antenatal and Postnatal Depression: Practical Advice and Support for All Sufferers*. London: Vermillion, p. 72.

29 Rosenfeld, D. (2006) ibid.

30 Cited in Wainwright, D. (1996) The political transformation of the health inequalities debate. *Critical Social Policy*, 16: 67–82.

31 Lee, C. and Owens, R.G. (2002) *The Psychology of Men's Health*. Buckingham: Open University Press, p. 3.

32 Leary, C. (n.d) Men's health: worth talking about. Available at: http://www.sanitarium.com.au

33 Connell, R.W. (1995) *Masculinities*. Cambridge: Polity; Horrocks, R. (1994) *Masculinity in Crisis: Myths, Fantasies and Realities*. London: Macmillan.

34 Royal College of Psychiatrists (2004), *Men Behaving Sadly*. Available on line at www.rcpsych.ac.uk

35 Fitzpatrick, M. (2006) The men's health movement: a morbid symptom. *Journal of Men's Health and Gender*, 3(3): 258–62.

36 Meryn, S. (2005) Men's Health 2005: A small step for mankind. *Journal of Men's Health and Gender*, 2(4): 389–90.

37 Gunnell, C. (2004) Do we know how to help men? *Community Practitioner*, 77(6): 204–5; White, E. (2004) Men's health: the hard facts. *Community Practitioner*, 77(6): 206–7.

38 Sontag, S. (1978) *Illness as Metaphor*. New York: Farrar, Strauss and Giroux.

39 Ehrenreich, B. (2001) Welcome to cancerland: a mammogram leads to a cult of pink kitsch. *Harper's Magazine* (November).

40 Olson, J. (2002) *Bathsheba's Breast: Women, Cancer and History*. Baltimore, MD: Johns Hopkins University Press, p. 127.

41 Olson, J. (2002) ibid., p. 108.

42 Breast cancer care (c. 2006) *Same Difference : Breast awareness is for everyone*. Available on line at www.breastcancer care.org.uk

43 Semiglazov, V.F., Moiseyenko, V.M., Bavli, J.L., Migmanova, N.S., Seleznyov, N.K., Popova, R.T., Ivanova, O.A., Orlov, A.A., Chagunava, O.A. and Barash, N.J. (1992) The role of breast self-examination in early breast cancer detection (results of the 5-year USSR/WHO randomised study in Leningrad). *European Journal of Epidemiology*, 8: 498–502; Thomas, D.B., Gao, D.L., Ray, R.M., Wang, W.W., Allison, C.J., Chen, F.L., Porter, P., Hu, Y.W., Zhao, G.L., Pan, L.D., Li, W., Wu, C., Coriaty, Z., Evans, I., Lin, M.G., Stalsberg, H. and Self, S.G. (2002) Randomised trial of breast self-examination in Shanghai: final results. *Journal of National Cancer Institute*, 94: 1445–57.

44 Gøtzsche, P.C. and Nielsen, M. (2006) *Screening for breast cancer with mammography*. Cochrane Database of Systematic Reviews, Issue 4.

45 Thornton, H., Edwards, A. and Baum, M. (2003) Women need better information about routine mammography. *British Medical Journal*, 327: 101–3.

46 Slaytor, E.K. and Ward, J.E. (1998) How risks of breast cancer and benefits of screening are communicated to women: analysis of 58 pamphlets. *British Medical Journal*, 317: 263–4.

47 Breast cancer care, ibid, p. 1.

48 Moore, S. (2006) PhD thesis, University of Kent. 'Ribbon wearing: a socio-cultural investigation'.

49 Carlowe, J. (2004) Boys don't cry. *Observer,* 10 October.
50 McCartney, M. (2004) Screening must remain a free choice. *British Medical Journal,* 328: 1023.
51 Coley, C.M., Barry, M.J., Fleming, C. and Mulley, A.J. (1997) Early detection of prostate cancer: part 1: Prior probability and effectiveness of tests. *Annals of Internal Medicine,* 126(5): 394–406.
52 Tannock, I. (2002) Eradication of a disease: how we cured symptomless prostate cancer. *The Lancet,* 359:1341–2.
53 Prostate Cancer Charity (2006) Product information. Available at: http://www.prostate-cancer.org.uk/
54 Fitzpatrick, M. (2001) ibid., p. 64.
55 Wainwright, D. (1996) ibid., p. 79.

8

Medicine, Science and 'Higher Superstition'

Tracey Brown

- Medical science represents the highest achievement of the Enlightenment project, freeing humanity from many of the worst excesses of nature.
- The Evidence-Based Medicine movement which emerged over the last 30 years should be the final step in the process of ensuring that medical practice is determined by the highest standards of scientific rigour, but just as this principle was established an anti-scientific backlash began.
- The 'science wars' were fought by a loose aggregation of post-modernists, feminists and 'complementary therapists' against what they saw as the scientific establishment.
- The war may be over, but the 'peace settlement' has left the scientific community in a defensive mood, grappling with new institutional arrangements which aim to 'democratise' science but may impede its progress.

Nature is dumb. In vain appeal to it.

Voltaire (1694–1778) *Poem on the Lisbon Disaster*

The relationship between science and medicine has never been straightforward. It has taken more than two centuries for the aspiration to understand – and then to heal – the human body to be translated into effective, systematic medical intervention based on clinical science. It is, though, fair to characterise the trajectory of modernity as being a halting move towards science and evidence as the basis of how medicine is practised. Scientific medicine, as part of science more generally, has been central to aspirations for social progress.

More prosaically, today there is an expectation widely held among the public that the treatment choices offered through modern health care services are based on scientific evidence, independently reviewed and regulated. In Anglo-American cultures particularly, if doctors do not adhere to accepted standards of practice and treatment they are liable to action for redress through the civil courts, disciplinary action by professional regulatory bodies and even criminal prosecution. In all modern societies, the licensing of medicines is expected to be rigorously scientific.

According to the Food and Drug Administration, which regulates medicines in the United States: since the early part of the last century, the public's basic expectations have been that all marketed drugs should be effective and safe within the context of their use and that unsafe or ineffective drugs should be kept off the market.[1]

In the UK, the central role of scientific research and clinical evidence in medicine was instituted through the Medicines Act 1968, which established strict controls on the marketing of drugs and devices, through independent review of clinical and toxicological data and routine surveillance for adverse drug reactions (side effects). Similar legislation is now in place across most parts of the world. While it is unlikely that the wider public is familiar with the specific details of drug approval or professional standards, social surveys and patient research suggest that the public expects medicine to be guided by scientific evidence.[2] If anything, expectations of the role of science in medicine are unrealistically high: one British poll shows that 61 per cent of the public expects science to give 100 per cent guarantees about the safety of medicines.[3] General medical practitioners regularly achieve the highest scores in surveys on public confidence in different professions.

However, the very dominance of scientific medicine appears to have created a 'backlash'. Despite the public's expectations of science, and the battles won to establish its importance among the medical professions, since the 1990s there has been a growing social inclination towards unorthodox, unproven treatments and alternative sources of medical and scientific authority. Remedies and practices marketed as traditional or 'natural' are held to offer alternatives to the 'drugs or do nothing' culture that is pejoratively ascribed to modern medicine. At the same time, there is also popular interest in new ideas for which there is little scientific support or no evidence that they work, that is, their *efficacy*, particularly in relation to chronic, poorly understood or untreatable conditions. There is a more diffuse but related development in the growth of a lifestyle sector around health claims that purport to be scientifically based, offering cures and protection against disease through a wide range of diets and lifestyle routines. Many of these dispute mainstream scientific views.

Arguments for *Evidence-Based Medicine* are challenged by these new claims for alternative outlooks and remedies. Unlike the popular challenges of the past, many of the unorthodox, unproven claims are presented not in ignorance of the science, but either in spite of it or in quasi-scientific terms. It is not expected that they will be invalidated by evidence in the way that traditions, beliefs and superstitions have been previously, because their essential proposition is that they are an *alternative* to medicine driven by mainstream scientific research or even a strong reaction against it. The argument put forward in support is that to deny equal status to these alternatives is to deny patient choice or to protect unreasonably the dominance of the medical establishment.

This challenge to the *hegemony* of scientific medicine is occurring in the context of broader questioning of the nature of science itself. Some of this is directed at the prestige and authority enjoyed by scientific institutions and at the power of large industries, particularly the pharmaceutical industry, which is accused of maintaining particular, scientifically supported outlooks that protect vested interests. It is pointed out that scientific discoveries have led to destructive technologies and that serious medical error and socially abhorrent practices have been conducted under the dominions of science. So while expectations of Evidence-Based Medicine are high, there is a growing social emphasis on the imperfect nature of scientific knowledge and the dangers of its authority, especially in the context of a doctor–patient relationship.

There are also more fundamental, ideological disputes about the assumption, associated with the Enlightenment, that the application of human reason to the laws of nature leads to social progress. Some social and cultural critics of science confine themselves to highlighting the limits of what is or can be scientifically known, urging a more humble approach to the gains that are claimed, for example, concerning the human genome or the safety of anti-viral drugs. However, science has become the subject of more systematic criticism for its claims to objectivity. Scientifically observed phenomena, it is argued, are no more 'true' or valuable than other forms of knowledge such as folklore or personal perception. Science – especially scientific medicine – has no place ridiculing other kinds of knowledge about the natural world when it is itself a social construct, reflecting and reinforcing its own traditions and orthodoxies, its vested interests and self-perpetuating processes. This constructivist outlook now informs, to varying degrees, the majority of academic discussion about science across sociology, cultural studies and philosophy. In a well-known critique of their popularity, these ideas have been described by the North American science writers Paul Gross and Norman Levitt as a kind of 'higher superstition'.[4]

There seem to be a number of different causes for a backlash. Indeed there is more than one backlash, which is explored in the sections that follow. But they all push in the same direction, away from science and scientific medicine, and they appear to be having a mutually reinforcing impact on social values and scientific institutions. Scientific and medical professionals have found it difficult to promote Evidence-Based Medicine against express disregard for the value of accumulated knowledge. They perceive the inadequacy of insisting on facts and evidence in a context where the status of facts and evidence – indeed the very existence of these things – is called into question. Where Gross and Levitt used 'higher superstition' to refer to the intellectual assault, we might characterise the combined backlash as wilful superstition. As modern societies move towards an increasing, practical dependence on evidence for the delivery of effective health care, locating the basis of the relationship between science and medicine has, ironically, never been so challenging.

The Evidence-Based Medicine movement

Evidence-Based Medicine has been most usefully defined as 'the conscientious, explicit, judicious use of current best evidence in making decisions about the care of individual patients'.[5] This definition should be noted for its emphasis on care of individual patients, because Evidence-Based Medicine is now frequently caricatured by its critics as paying no attention to patients' needs and reducing them to study statistics or drug consumers. With the growth of alternative medicine and conflict over knowledge and medical practice, it is helpful to reprise some key aspects of the relationship between medicine and science.

For more than three decades, there has been a concerted movement among the medical establishment – the professions, health care providers, drug manufacturers and medical research – towards insisting that the impact of medical interventions on the course of disease should be demonstrated empirically. Medicine was the first area in which there were attempts to assimilate systematically evidence from scientific research into policy decisions. From today's standpoint, where expectations of efficacy and safety are high in mainstream medicine, it may not be immediately obvious why Evidence-Based Medicine should have required a concerted movement to become established.

The application of scientific research methods to medicine has a long history. To 'first do no harm' practitioners must be familiar with the likely outcome of their interventions and this implies a respect for evidence. But a willingness to respond to evidence did not translate directly into obtaining that evidence – through the systematic application of scientific principles to observations – and bringing it to bear on medical practice. To do this required both the possibility of conducting such research (something which was only possible with the advent of modern healthcare among other things) and an effort of will to organise it. Awareness of such clinical data as did exist and the insights that could be generated through reviewing it and identifying questions for clinical research developed slowly until the late 1960s.

This is not to say that safety, efficacy and professional standards were new concerns: they had been regulated in a variety of ways in the majority of developed countries for over a century. Indeed, the 1968 Medicines Act in the UK drew together assorted regulations, legislation and other measures that had been introduced in response to problems and inconsistencies in the way that medicine was practised. These previous efforts had brought medicine closer to science as the chief means of raising standards and effectiveness, often bringing their supporters into collision with traditional practices. However, they had proved insufficient. The Act was, in large part, a response to an investigation of the widespread use of thalidomide as an anti-emetic drug for pregnant women in the 1950s and 1960s. The effects of the drug on foetal development had not been researched and only became clear when nearly 12,000 children had been born with severe limb deformities in those countries where thalidomide was licensed. The deficiencies in the testing and licensing regimes were not the only problem revealed by this tragedy. The lack of a centralised system for reporting adverse incidents meant that health care professionals had attributed the deformities to a range of factors that appeared to them, locally, to be likely. Those who noted the drug as a common factor were unable to report or compare their concerns quickly. The scale of the damage caused helped to turn everyone's attention to the need for safety data, efficacy testing, and risk/benefit assessments through rigorous licensing, prescribing and reporting rules. Today, the thalidomide incident is often cited to contradict positive views of the role of modern medicine in progress. It is worth noting that at the time, while some of the popular commentary challenged medical science, the thalidomide incident was handled by official bodies not as a failure of science but as a failure of the regulation of medicines and as indicating a greater need for science.

In 1972, the pioneering document on evidence in medicine, *Effectiveness and Efficiency*,[6] was published in the UK by Archie Cochrane, whose name was later given to the collaboration centre in Oxford, UK, which now leads an international programme of systematic reviews on the effectiveness of health care interventions. This document set out the need for data collection and review to establish which treatments worked and which did not. With this attempt to address more directly the task of gradually reviewing all existing practices, and keeping new ones under surveillance, the Evidence-Based Medicine movement began.

Why is scientific evidence not a straightforward matter in medicine? In large part it is because subjective clinical observations are often compelling. In deciding which treatments are working or not, both clinicians and patients are affected by inclinations, wishful thinking and despondency. These can have a very powerful effect on how a treatment is administered and taken, and what its effects are perceived to be. The gap between perception, even across whole communities of practitioners, and clinical evidence can be very large, with the evidence seeming to be highly counterintuitive. For example, tonsillectomy has been widely practised in cases of recurring tonsillitis in children. It has shocked many general practitioners, surgeons and patients to learn that the longer-term outcomes (six months to two years) are the same for those that don't have the procedure as for those that do, but without the risks of surgery.

The only way to discover the true effects of an intervention is in a fair test and one where the role of bias and the play of chance can be ruled out (or near to it). There are several effective methods for doing this depending on the nature of the question being investigated.[7] In respect of the debates about scientific medicine and the backlash against it, it is particularly worth commenting on three: double blinding, randomisation and cumulative reviews.

A trial is *double blind* when neither the person administering the treatment nor the patient know whether they are getting the actual treatment or an identical-looking placebo such as a pill without the active ingredient. Double-blind tests help to show whether changes in a condition are actually attributable to the specific procedure or to something else like time spent with a doctor. If wishful thinking and other attitudes can play a strong role in actual health outcomes (placebo effect) and in reported outcomes then it is easy to see how interventions based on different belief systems, such as homeopathy, might be particularly prone to these biases.

Another significant way that results of studies can be biased is in the selection of people being studied. For this reason, clinical trials are usually *randomised* – that is, the test population is randomly assigned to the groups receiving the treatment and those receiving the placebo. This is frequently confused in popular commentary with a 'random selection' of people, such as consumers who have used a product, which does not have the effect of removing bias from the findings.

Finally, Evidence-Based Medicine is emphatically cumulative. It is well recognised that individual studies can produce misleading results, perhaps because of chance, especially if they are conducted with small samples, and perhaps because they were not designed in a way that eliminated biases. It is for this reason that the popular appearance of many therapeutic areas is of a constant flow of media reports that contradict each other. One month a study shows that a chemical may cause breast cancer; the next a large epidemiological study shows that it is unlikely to be a factor. Similarly, a class of drugs called statins are shown in some studies to be a 'wonder drug' to reduce heart attacks, but then are said to have little effect on many patients. Through reviewing all the studies of a particular condition or intervention, it is more likely that consistent patterns of benefits and risks are identified and it is often possible to decide where, overall, the weight of evidence lies much more reliably. Reviews of new data in the light of existing data also help to assimilate what has already been demonstrated and to eliminate a lot of unnecessary research, thereby reducing exposure to risks and delays in effective treatment.

In terms of the old struggle against inertia and tradition, the insights and improvements gained through Evidence-Based Medicine have decisively won support. Tensions between the practice of medicine and clinical science do still occur, particularly when long-established practices are challenged by scientific reviews that fail to show any benefits from them. This was notable in the discovery that breast cancer patients undergoing radical mastectomy (complete removal of both breasts) did not have better outcomes than patients undergoing the much less traumatic procedure of localised tissue removal and radiotherapy.[8] There is also, necessarily, a lag between new scientific findings and their adoption so these tensions will never be entirely overcome. But the role of evidence and scientific trials is now central to medicine, supported morally, empirically and through legislation. As a review of the international situation has commented:

> Although there is still some resistance to the evidence-based medicine movement, evidence-based health care has now become widely accepted and adopted. Systematic reviews of the effectiveness of health care interventions are the engine room of evidence-based health care.[9]

Ideological challenges

Does medical science 'know' what's best for us?

Where the Evidence-Based Medicine movement encouraged a rigorous questioning of the evidential basis for medical practice, the question, 'How do you know it works?' is now being used in a different, rhetorical way that suggests suspicion rather than inquiry. There is a growing interest in beliefs and practices that do not reflect the contemporary understanding of human physiology and which tend to base their authority on tradition rather than on scientific evidence that they work. These include acupuncture, chiropractic, herbalism, osteopathy and homeopathy, which are generally referred to as the 'big five' alternative traditions. Although little social research has been conducted into how widespread or frequent use of alternative medicines is, their popularity is implied by the multi-million pound industries that now manufacture and sell them in the UK and in most other European countries. Despite their incompatibility with scientific medicine, they are increasingly promoted as 'complementary' systems that should be given the same support as Evidence-Based Medicine.

There is considerable debate about whether clinical trials might find that some alternative treatments are efficacious. While the dilutions of homeopathic medicines are so great that the chances of a molecule of active ingredient being present in the pills is smaller than winning the lottery several weeks in a row, it is much more likely that some herbal medicines could have an effect on the course of disease. Indeed, regulatory authorities are considering their possible effects with concern following reports of herbal medicines interfering in the effects of blood clotting drugs and cancer treatments. Many medical scientists argue that there are not different kinds of medicine – just medicine that works and 'medicine' that does not. Proof of efficacy would make these alternatives part of mainstream medicine. This is consistent with the approach of the Evidence-Based Medicine movement. However, the attraction of alternative medicine seems to be that it is *not* part of mainstream medicine. Moreover, advocates of alternative medicine often argue that it defies the kind of clinical study that is called for by scientific medicine. As Adam Wishart has noted in his account of his father's cancer treatment, 'Although there were many different schools of alternative medicine, ranging from the use of ancient herbs to mind-over-body techniques, its therapists ... subscribed to a similar critique of orthodox medicine'.[10] It is this search for an alternative that poses some challenging questions about the social dynamics around medicine today.

The search for alternatives to scientific medicine is not confined to the resurrection of traditional beliefs over evidence, as in the cases of homeopathy and herbalism. Some groups who reject orthodox medicine reject the medical paradigm. The natural childbirth movement is hostile to the medicalisation of pregnancy and childbirth, where women are monitored by medical professionals throughout pregnancy and the majority of births are expected to take place in hospitals, many with medical assistance. Proponents argue for a rejection of this 'scientistic' approach. Similarly, the anti-vaccination movements that have been so prominent in campaigns against the Measles Mumps Rubella (MMR) vaccine are not necessarily advocates of alternative medicine but reject the intervention and are not swayed by the evidence. In some part this was a reaction to the patient's experience of medical care, particularly of surgery and hospitalisation – experiences which are often found to be disempowering. Social theorists have argued that an infantilising dynamic is central to the current models of health care, which take as their starting point the superior knowledge of professionals.

These movements remain at the margins of society but they do seem to respond to a more undefined but widespread frustration with mainstream medicine. Medical advances have not led to effective responses to the challenges of diseases such as cancer and AIDS and have little to offer for many chronic diseases. Where the benefits of scientific medicine in earlier interventions had been more straightforward and self-evident, few of the conditions that challenge medical science today are resolved so decisively. Certainly, there seems to be some indication that rejection of scientific medicine has historically been subsumed in decisive advances. The anti-vaccination movement began in the 1850s following the introduction of a compulsory vaccine against smallpox in 1853. In the UK it was managed, but not resolved, with introduction of a 'conscientious objection' clause just before the First World War. However, uptake was sufficient and the subsequent eradication of smallpox, along with the benefits of the typhoid vaccine for troops fighting in the trenches in the First World War, helped to ensure that vaccination was looked on positively and as a social responsibility. Some people argue that by contrast today we have little collective memory of the devastating impact of diseases such as measles and we almost never, in modern European societies, see cases of rubella-damaged babies.

The currently intractable problems of incurable diseases and chronic conditions do appear to be responsible for a lot of interest in alternative treatments. There is also a growth in symptom-led conditions that are experienced as medical but for which scientific medicine has no diagnosis much less a therapeutic response. In combination, these have created a market for health outside of the traditional health care practitioner relationship. Popular commentary relating health to lifestyle, food and environment has grown enormously in the past ten years, together with increased TV coverage and the expanding World Wide Web, to respond to this market. In the daily newspapers too, lifestyle columns, supplements and health advice fight news content for space.

Responses to this demand for something more than scientific medicine can often include not just the appeal to tradition of alternative medicine, but also greater interest in quasi-scientific avant-garde medicine. This is theories and remedies that purport to be based on science that is as yet unrecognised by the medical establishment. It is sometimes argued that particular social forces dominate mainstream medical research and that advocates of Evidence-Based Medicine are too blinkered or too self-preserving to recognise new insights:

> The Cochrane Group, among others, has created a hierarchy that has been endorsed by many academic institutions, and that serves to (re)produce the exclusion of certain forms of research. Because 'regimes of truth' such as the evidence-based movement currently enjoy a privileged status, scholars have not only a scientific duty, but also an ethical obligation to deconstruct these regimes of power.[11]

In a more diffuse form of this argument, scientific knowledge and the desire for medical progress are associated with corruption and private interest. It is argued that the medical establishment, perhaps including drug companies, uses demands for scientific evidence as a system for suppressing innovation and discovery. This outlook is supported by an alternative health care industry whose marketing and publicity materials reflect contemporary ambivalence about the idea that orthodox medicine 'knows best'.

The more equivocal idea about the limits of medicine has been, in part, responsible for defensiveness among the medical professions. In their turn, they have been less inclined to resist some of the criticism and in some cases have found common cause with attacks on the 'doctor knows best' idea that has become a shorthand reference to the confidence of the professions in the past. There is considerable irony that alternative medicine presents itself as ranged against the resistance and closed-mindedness that have in earlier times been a challenge for the Evidence-Based Medicine movement. However, this movement now finds itself accused of the same for its very insistence on evidence and science.

Another irony is to be found in the presentation of alternative medicine as offering a more 'holistic' approach. If modern medicine has moved with science towards an evidence-based approach, it has also maintained a holistic approach based on personal appointments and whole-person appraisal. The definition given at the beginning of this section, with the emphasis on the individual patient, is the one that is commonly ascribed to. At its simplest level, this is reflected in prescribing behaviour among general practitioners taking into account personal circumstances and likely compliance with treatment. For example, it is recognised that the ability of a patient to comply with a treatment regime that involves taking a prescribed medicine three times a day, after meals, at regular intervals varies enormously between a stable middle-class, middle-aged woman and a homeless young man with alcohol addiction. In practice, however, doctors are often frustrated by the lack of resources available.

The science wars

The rise of wilful superstition, generated from the standpoint of frustration with or hostility to scientific medicine rather than in ignorance of it, calls into question the value that societies ascribe to accumulated knowledge and the entitlements to authority that knowledge bestows. But this is only an implication of the turn to alternatives and is usually made explicit only pragmatically, in order to create the space for an alternative to be advanced. In academic debate, however, there has been a much more sustained and pointed attack on science and scientific knowledge claims.

This attack has coincided with a general loss of confidence across advanced modern societies in the idea that science delivers progress. Without the optimism that had been associated with advances in scientific knowledge and application – for their contribution to challenging traditional authority and human suffering – the scientific world now appeared to be enjoying unwarranted influence and power. Some criticism started out as a reaction to the apparent 'clubiness' and complacency of science. From the late 1980s, the academic critique of scientific rationality has gained momentum. Scientific knowledge, it is contended, is not free from the values and influences within which it is generated; it is socially constructed. The development of *social constructivism* has moved towards a rejection of the notion of objective observation. Some social constructivists argue that scientific observations of the natural world are no more inherently 'true' than other perceptions or forms of knowledge such as folklore. If that is so, on what authority do scientists pronounce on others' ideas or influence policy or enjoy social status? One answer to this question is provided by cultural theory, which is more emphatic that scientific knowledge is itself little more than a tool of power and control and that, consciously or unconsciously, it has developed to reinforce the domination of powerful elites, of men over women and of white professionals over other ethnic and social groups.

These are, largely, not responses to specific experiences or scientific claims but are more of a political attack on science as a way of knowing, as a body of knowledge and as the means of wielding power. They represent something of a triumph for Foucault's concept of knowledge as power. The debates that have ensued, about the nature of knowledge and the claims of science, are referred to as the 'Science Wars'.

The 'Science Wars', taken in their own terms, appear as an intellectual debate, and one that has frequently been presented in caricatures, with positivistic, arrogant scientists on the one hand and post-modern social scientists who hold that nothing is true and science is just a cultural construct on the other. While the arguments are provocative and worth examining in their own terms, what is of greater significance is the broader shift in attitudes to accumulated knowledge and scientific endeavour that occurred alongside them and which have interacted with critiques of science at intellectual and pragmatic levels.

This is somewhat different from the way in which science was disparaged earlier in the twentieth century. When C.P. Snow famously wrote about the 'two cultures' – scientific and literary – in 1959, the debate was about the social value that we place on art and on science.[12] Science deals with the facts, it was argued, not with what is beautiful or desirable. Although arguments continue about the cultural importance of science, it is the assertion of objectivity that is at issue today.

The term *post-modernism* is used quite commonly today to refer to what would be more accurately described as social constructivism and varying degrees of relativism. In the 1980s, post-modernism, in its strict sense, enjoyed some short-lived popularity in the humanities and to a lesser extent in the social sciences. It seemed to capture a moment when people became more alienated from social institutions and from mainstream sources of authority, by emphasising the fragmentary nature of experience. The post-modern idea was, really, just an assertion and, in the absence of a strong intellectual framework, some post-modernist thinkers drew for credibility on concepts in the physical sciences that suggested disorder at the heart of the universe. Scientific inquiry was dismissed by post-modernism – implicitly and explicitly – but this made little impact on wider attitudes and the superficial links that some writers drew between social relations and natural laws collapsed under the minimum of scrutiny. In fact, contrary to current assumptions, many social constructivists and cultural theorists were hostile to the implicit suggestion of post-modernist philosophers that meaning was generated randomly, independent of social relations. To accept this proposition would in effect render any kind of social action or critique – or science – pointless.

It was in the early 1990s that social constructivism began to take hold in the discussion of science and that 'science studies' emerged as an academic discipline. The target of objections from early representatives of science studies were the 'truth claims' made for science. Although they were not ostensibly motivated by an attack on the large-scale expenditure on big science projects that had been associated with the Cold War, it is likely that they gained more ground because they coincided with a dampening of political (and financial) commitment to such projects.

The science world has a high representation of men and has drawn some of its most fervent criticism from feminist thinkers within social constructivism. In part, these are arguments for inclusion. Sandra Harding, who allegedly claimed that Isaac Newton's *Principia Mathematica* is a 'rape manual' because 'science is a male rape of female nature',[13] stresses the significance of women's perceptions and analysis, arguing that they have value in scientific and technological work. This perspective, known as feminist standpoint theory, has not been widely advanced however. The more frequent argument made is that science is subject to social forces, as advanced by another feminist theorist: 'on every level, choices are made – of what it is that we want to know, of how we ought to proceed, of what counts as knowledge – and these choices are social even as they are cognitive and experimental'.[14]

Empirical studies are rarely called upon. Indeed, much of the constructivist assertion about science lacks even anecdotal support. However, the view that scientific knowledge represents just one kind of 'knowing' and there are other discourses, such as those based on personal experiences or stories, which should be viewed as no less important in generating knowledge, has been more widely attractive for its appearance of being democratic. Advocates argue that we should stop treating expert knowledge as privileged.

Throughout the science wars, many arguments have been advanced against the social constructivist view of knowledge, by both left and right, from within science and from other quarters. That science is not itself democratic – we do not decide what is most likely to be true by voting on it – does not mean that scientists are anti-democratic. Scientific knowledge is different from socially agreed norms. A leading writer on the history of science, John Gribbin, has argued that, contrary to the views of some sociologists and historians, scientific truth cannot be equated with artistic truth. Rather, science is to some extent divorced from the economic and social upheavals going on in the world at large, and it is a search for objective truth.[15] This is an argument that is difficult to dispute. The law of gravity was the same for the Incas as it is in modern-day Japan. Society's relationship to it has changed – we now manipulate the laws of nature, such as with skyscrapers, elevators and aeroplanes.

Thoughtful critics of the constructivist school have sought to make the distinction between what they would regard as a legitimate approach to the institutions of science, which are social, and science itself.[16] This distinction became clearer in a row about the nature of knowledge claims following a hoax perpetrated by a left-wing scientist in order to expose the constructivist school.

Sokal's hoax

The science wars are now considered by many to have peaked in the mid-1990s following the exposure of 'Sokal's hoax', which became a symbol of the science wars. The hoax is a useful window on the frustrations of the 'science wars' arguments. In 1994, Alan Sokal, a professor of physics at New York University, set out to expose the growing fashion for the cultural and constructivist theories of science and what he regarded as their pretensions to substantial analysis in the place where critical analysis should be clearest. He wrote an article called 'Transgressing the boundaries: towards a transformative hermeneutics of quantum gravity', in which he purported to argue that the laws of nature are socially constructed. Throughout the article, he inserted, often at random, phrases in vogue among the cultural theorists:

> It has thus become increasingly apparent that physical "reality", no less than social "reality", is at bottom a social and linguistic construct; that scientific "knowledge", far from being objective, reflects and encodes the dominant ideologies and power relations of the culture that produced it; that the truth claims of science are inherently theory-laden and self-referential; and consequently, that the discourse of the scientific community, for all its undeniable value, cannot assert a privileged epistemological status with respect to counter-hegemonic narratives emanating from dissident or marginalized communities.[17]

Sokal submitted this satirical article to the cultural studies journal *Social Text*, whose editors failed to realise that it was a hoax and published it in the Spring/Summer 1996 issue. Sokal then immediately published his exposé of his hoax in another journal, in which he criticised the editors of *Social Text* for publishing an article on quantum physics without feeling the need to consult anyone who knew about the subject. He accused the editors of being so flattered by the use of terms of which they approved that they had willingly published his 'self-indulgent nonsense'.[18]

The author's revelation of his hoax provoked a very angry response from the cultural theorists. The editors of *Social Text* argued, in their defence, that they had not understood the science and that they had published the essay because it dovetails with post-modern theory. Several commentators on this incident pointed out that this was Sokal's point: to expose the pretensions of the cultural theorists to understand what they most disparaged, but more importantly to expose the laziness and muddled thinking of much constructivist discourse in science studies. Sokal was not so much trying to defend science with this hoax, although he is frustrated by insubstantial critiques, as to draw the attention of the Left to its own 'disastrous thinking'.

The weakening of constructivist approaches to science

The row about the Sokal hoax was not just a debate that animated the academic sides of the science wars. Newspapers and magazines internationally covered the story and it became the focal point for a critical discussion about the state of cultural studies of science. In particular, the publication of the hoax piece drew strong criticism from others on the academic Left who did not take a post-modern, relativist or extreme constructivist approach to knowledge. Subsequently, the cultural critique of science has lost much of its academic force. Whether as a result of the criticism and embarrassment from within the social sciences and humanities, or because the approach seems to have failed to deliver a coherent critique of scientific knowledge and expertise, is a matter of ongoing debate.

What is very likely is that that driving force for the constructivist argument – the frustration with the influence of science – has lost some of the momentum of the initial, quite dramatic loss of confidence in scientific progress in the 1980s and 1990s. Second, while attacking knowledge has created some considerable space for alternative sources of authority and expertise in public life, science has not made a particularly good target for challenging power relations. It necessitates undermining knowledge as the basis for objecting to inequality and it undermines the possibility that the human condition could be improved practically through medicine, public health and new technologies. As several commentators on the science wars have pointed out, powerful elites have the guns and money, why should radical critics cede to them clear thinking too?

Under these pressures, the constructivist argument retreats into pointing out human fallibility and inconsistencies in the application of scientific principles or use of evidence. The fallibility of science is regularly highlighted in discussions about alternative sources of knowledge. In this way, it is used to suggest that all things qualify as legitimate. However, this sets up scientific knowledge as something of a straw man, suggesting that it makes claims of certainty and infallibility that are not in evidence. As the commentator James Robert Brown argues, 'scientific objectivity is compatible with a high degree of fallibility'.[19]

A further weakness in the constructivist appeal is that their reaction to scientific 'control' of knowledge is to promote the authority of other kinds of knowledge or expertise. In this sense, it is simply copying what it criticises, and establishing expertise as a route to power and authority. Not surprisingly, the beneficiaries of this new expert space have been a small, elite group of critics and some campaigners who have adopted their successful innovation of opening up space for influence by making traditional authorities defensive. It has created a pattern for others who want to make a bid for authority and managerial influence, but one that, while arguably as exclusive, removes the knowledge relationship with the wider population.

The direct assertion that knowledge is a social or cultural construct has also been difficult for its advocates to sustain on a more practical basis in modern societies where we depend on our houses being wired for electricity and where we expect heart bypass operations to extend life. In those conditions, the view that nothing is known and that all discourses are equally valid is likely to strike many people as fatuous. However, as we see in the following section, while the realities of modern social and political existence constrain the ideological attack, they also are unable to resist it in parts. In a more popular form, weakened versions of constructivist ideas are proving irresistible as a possible constraint on the authority of science in a range of settings.

Defensive science: participation and democratisation

Beyond the heated exchanges of the science wars, which were often confined to college campuses of the United States, few scientists have found themselves equipped with a convincing reply to hostility and there has been little concerted resistance to the attacks on science and scientific medicine. Despite the weaknesses and contradictory character of challenges to scientific knowledge and evidence, many institutions have responded by embracing the demands for *'democratisation'*, lay involvement, expansion of experts and constraints on scientific research. While the science and the claims made by scientists have been presented in caricatured form in much of the debates about science and scientific medicine, the charges of arrogance and elitism have succeeded in making many scientific institutions defensive. Representatives of orthodox medicine have been particularly sensitive to criticism. This is probably in part because it is medical science that has so frequently been at issue and in part because clinical application dictates a closer connection with the public and it is therefore necessarily sensitive to social trends and public perceptions.

In surveys of public attitudes to professionals, doctors generally do well and are cited as one of the most trusted groups. However, this is not fully reflected in the way that patients behave. There is much reference to the 'end of a culture of deference' towards doctors and to the emergence of a 'second-opinion culture'. These are regularly discussed in popular commentary and in the pages of medical publications. The growth of alternatives to mainstream medicine implies a distrust or dissatisfaction. This inability to satisfy patients is keenly felt through the perceived threat of litigation, which also provokes much comment among the medical professions as well as leading to the implementation of new codes designed to avoid misunderstandings and recriminations.

There is another argument that supports the institutionalisation of lay committees to review scientific decisions. It is argued that science – particularly medical science – is now moving so fast and transgressing boundaries that have substantively bigger ethical implications. In particular, gene technologies and stem cell research are cited. This view sees the opportunity for lay review and input from other kinds of experts as a welcome constraint on scientific research and technological innovation that might otherwise introduce unwanted fundamental changes in our existence.

Individuals from government, academia and the civic sector who lead the challenges to scientific authority have flattered cynical attitudes to expertise, elevating subjective, intuitive responses. Their cause has often been presented in aggressively populist terms, sometimes as a 'grassroots' request for empowerment. Populism is difficult to resist without appearing to endorse arrogance or elitism. In effect, a trap is laid whereby insistence on scientific evidence or attachment to medical expertise is equated with a desire to return to a lost age of deference and 'doctor knows best'.

Health care practitioners and scientists are also inhibited by their own awareness of the fallibility of medical science and limits of current knowledge. As discussed earlier, effective therapeutic responses to AIDS and many cancers have been elusive. Improvements in drugs for chronic conditions have happened, but they have tended to be incremental and not on the scale of innovation or eradication of suffering associated with vaccines, hip replacements or heart transplants. Many scientists are also uncomfortable with the politically driven agenda for science and with the lack of measure in claims that national governments have made from the 'war against cancer' of the Nixon years to the idea of economic recovery through the 'biotechnology revolution' today. In such circumstances, even the consensus about the dramatic gains of medical science of the past is more readily questioned. Earlier arguments that, contrary to received wisdom, improvements in life expectancy and health came about largely through public health measures[20] are being redeployed to this debate about the desirability of scientific medicine.

A further cause of defensiveness in medical science is the public hostility to the power and influence of the pharmaceutical industry. This hostility has had little impact on demands for both prescription and over-the-counter medicines, but it is widely articulated through the media internationally, and it is expressed through popular culture too. Sectors and companies have become by-words for corporate power, 'Big Tobacco', 'Big Pharma', Monsanto and Exxon are common examples. As many articles in the pages of the *British Medical Journal*, the *Journal of the American Medical Association* and other medical publications point out, the research agenda is shaped by political and commercial funding priorities. Anxiety about vested interests in scientific medicine has become firmly entrenched in the professional, as well as the popular, sphere.

The approach of pointing to shortcomings in processes to call into question general principles is particularly strong in the discussion about the shortcomings of the peer-review system. That scientific journals have published papers with substantial flaws, or rejected those with scientific merit, or that the system, like any reliance on human judgement and trust, can be found wanting, few would deny. This is a kind of chastening thesis – the seeking of agreement that scientific medicine is not so impressive – from which point it becomes easier to advance the inclusion of alternative experts and new layers of managerial constraint. Doctors and scientists are themselves sometimes attracted to this kind of thesis because they too are aware of the potential for error and revision. It should be noted that there is not a discussion about the usefulness of having lay members on committees, or putting proposals to ethics groups, both of which have been used in the past by bodies who have found benefits from them. It is a discussion about entitlement and participation on a moral basis, for its own sake, as described in Sandra Harding's arguments for feminist standpoint theory.[21]

More significantly than these difficulties in resisting populist initiatives and chastening arguments, acceptance of them offers a kind of peace, whether from the science wars or from the unpleasant and disruptive attacks on scientific research, particular technologies and medicine. Research funders, government commissions and communications initiatives have urged this acceptance on their scientific constituencies, in an attempt at consensus building and for fear of losing public legitimacy. By redefining the backlash against scientific medicine and attacks on science into problems of scientific arrogance or lack of political consultation, they become manageable. In this activity, many different groups conspire in search of a more peaceful and pleasant arrangement. In the process, scientists fail to address the hostility and conceptions of science that inform the backlash.

The new etiquette

Despite the widespread expectation that medicine should be science based, there is a reaction against scientific medicine. At the popular level this takes the form of a search for alternative therapies and authorities. Having established the importance of scientific training as the basis for medical authority, society's relationship with that authority is often uneasy. Expectations of evidence-driven medicine coexist with hostility to orthodox medical practices and knowledge.

At the level of academic debate, there has been a retreat from the idea that science contributes to social justice and progress, and the social constructivist critique has extended to challenging rationality and the very possibility of scientific knowledge. Unlike the earlier challenges to evidence-based medicine of overcoming superstition and tradition, these new challenges have developed in spite of science rather than in ignorance of it.

At the level of institutional governance, this wilful superstition and the demand for democratisation have led to an embrace of new forms of expertise and a formal recognition of alternative therapeutic approaches. Since the early 1990s, it has become commonplace for critics to develop new etiquettes about the way in which science, and medicine specifically, should engage the public. Academic arguments about the need to privilege lay knowledge have achieved little popular circulation, but initiatives to incorporate a broader range of expertise into medical science are now widespread. A space for doing this has been created by the belief that interaction between scientific and medical bodies and the wider public is highly problematic or unsatisfactory.

This interaction has also, in the process of opening up medical science to a broader range of concerns, become more problematic. One of the problems that it creates is to make responsibility much more diffuse. When, for example, a review of the scientific research on the Measles Mumps Rubella (MMR) combined vaccine included the groups of parents who objected to the vaccine because of newspaper stories about a possible link with autism in children, it caused confusion about what the criteria were for conclusions in the resulting report. Similarly, in 2000, the UK's House of Lords Select Committee Report on complementary and alternative medicine was so dominated by finding compromises between opposing views that the standards being applied in the judgements and recommendations were varied and unclear. Unexpectedly, involvement of lay groups and a wider pool of non-scientific expertise has made the process by which decisions are reached more mystifying and therefore harder for communities to understand and respond to. There is also a tension between extending decision making about medical science and research funding on the one hand and a stronger desire for accountability among medical experts, which is frequently given expression in legal action by patients and consumers.

Conclusion

Contrary to the popular appearance of initiatives such as lay committees and patient expertise, many of these initiatives were led from the top by the institutions that they are viewed as challenging. They appear to have found an accommodation, but it is one that reproduces ambivalence about scientific medicine and undermines knowledge-based accountability. While intended to promote legitimacy and a more peaceful, manageable set of relationships, they have the effect of side-stepping the hostility and other causes of reaction against scientific medicine instead of confronting them. Some initiatives, particularly around the use of alternative therapies, proceed in awareness of their failure to address this. What appears as a backlash is in fact the coalescence of trends, which have consolidated around a number of successful arguments, all of which concern the dominance of science. It is defensiveness among institutions that has given these reactions a permanent operational presence and has turned them from transient complaints into well-crafted appeals for influence. Scientific medicine, and to some extent scientific institutions more widely, have institutionalised their own backlash. As a self-conscious concession to arguments that are not privately endorsed, this contributes to bad faith and further politicises science. The successes of the Evidence-Based Medicine movement make less sense to such a politicised debate.

148

Discussion topics

- Can complementary and alternative medicine be 'evidence based'?
- Explore the proposition that science is just another belief system.
- Can science be democratic?

Further reading

Brown, J.R. (2001) *Who Rules in Science? An Opinionated Account of the Wars.* Cambridge, MA: Harvard University Press.

James Robert Brown reaches beyond the caricatures of the Science Wars as a debate between Left and Right to examine the social and political impact of social constructionism, including a thorough and illuminating account of the Sokal hoax. He explains what is meant by the scientific method (Chapter 2) and goes on to explore the historical and contemporary philosophical debates about science and reason.

Evans, I., Thornton, H. and Chalmers, I. (2006) *Testing Treatments: Better Research for Better Healthcare.* London: The British Library.

This book is about how medical research is designed to produce fair and reliable evidence about the efficacy of treatments. Through case studies and historical accounts it explains the development of Evidence-Based Medicine and looks at the sometimes astonishing insights that clinical trials have generated about therapies that work and those that do not.

Levitt, N. (1999) *Prometheus Bedevilled: Science and the Contradictions of Contemporary Culture.* New Brunswick, NJ: Rutgers University Press.

Norman Levitt, mathematician, writer and veteran of the Science Wars, addresses the challenge posed by the academic Left's embrace of obscurantist intellectual trends. Through a review of debates from the repatriation of remains to the democratisation of science, he argues that what is at issue is the progressive aspiration to knowledge and objectivity and thereby accountability.

Tallis, R. (2004) *Hippocratic Oaths: Medicine and Its Discontents.* London: Atlantic Books.

Ray Tallis reviews and challenges the cultural ambivalence that has recently emerged around medical progress and expertise. He examines the attacks on medicine and medical practice from media scares, the growth of pseudo science, and the extension of political control over the medical profession.

References

1 US Food and Drug Administration (2006) A conversation about the FDA and drug regulation. In *From Test Tube to Patient: Protecting America's Health Through Human Drugs* (Special Report, *FDA Consumer Magazine*), January.
2 General Medical Council (2001) *Good Medical Practice: The Duties of a Doctor Registered with the General Medical Council.* London: GMC Publications.

3   MORI (2002) *Public Expects the Impossible from Science*. Available at http://www.mori.com/polls/2002/science.shtml.
4   Gross, P.R. and Levitt, N. (1994) *Higher Superstition: The Academic Left and Its Quarrels with Science*. Baltimore, MD: Johns Hopkins University Press.
5   Sackett, D.L., Rosenberg, W.M.C., Muir Gray, J.A., Haynes, R.B. and Richardson, W.S. (1996) Evidence based medicine: what it is and what it isn't. *British Medical Journal*, 312: 71–2.
6   Cochrane, A. (1972/1999) *Effectiveness and Efficiency: Random Reflections on Health Services*. London: Royal Society of Medicine Press.
7   Evans, I., Thornton, H. and Chalmers, I. (2006) *Testing Treatments: Better Research for Better Healthcare*. London: British Library.
8   Evans, I., Thornton, H. and Chalmers, I. (2006) ibid.
9   Chinnock, P., Siegfried, N. and Clarke, M. (2005) Is evidence-based medicine relevant to the developing world? *Public Library of Science Medicine*, 2(5): 107.
10 Wishart, A. (2006) *One in Three*. London: Profile Books, pp. 141–2.
11 Holmes, D., Murray, S., Perron, A. and Rail, G. (2006) Deconstructing the evidence-based discourse in health sciences: truth, power and fascism. *International Journal of Evidence Based Healthcare*, 4: 180.
12 Snow, C.P. (1959) *The Two Cultures and the Scientific Revolution* (Rede lectures, 1959). Cambridge: Cambridge University Press.
13 Harding, S. (1986) *The Science Question in Feminism*. Ithaca, NY: Cornell University Press, p. 264.
14 Keller, E.F. (1995) Science and its critics. *Academe*, 81: 11.
15 Gribbin, J. (2003) *Science: A History, 1543–2001*. London: Penguin, p. 614.
16 Brown, J.R. (2001) *Who Rules in Science? An Opinionated Account of the Wars*. Cambridge, MA: Harvard University Press.
17 Sokal, A.D. (1996) Transgressing the boundaries: towards a transformative hermeneutics of quantum gravity. *Social Text*, 46/47: 217–52.
18 Sokal, A.D. (1996) A physicist experiments with cultural studies. *Lingua Franca*, May/June: 62–4.
19 Brown, J.R. (2001) ibid., p. 20.
20 McKeown, T. (1979) *The Role of Medicine: Dream, Mirage or Nemesis*. Princeton, NJ: Princeton University Press.
21 Harding, S. (1986) ibid.

9

New Dimensions of Health Care Organisation

Mike Bury

- Britain's National Health Service is changing rapidly from a centrally managed and state provided system to a more pluralistic model which incorporates the private sector and managed competition.
- This transition has been accompanied by equally dramatic changes in the nature of the medical profession and the role of the patient and public in health care.
- The medical profession continues to enjoy a high degree of status and authority, but the traditional autonomy and self-regulation of the profession are increasingly challenged by managerialism, corporatisation, litigation, and a greater emphasis on regulation and accountability.
- The rationale for change is to make the NHS more responsive to the needs and preferences of patients and the public. The notion of a 'patient-led NHS' implies greater choice and control, but with this comes a new responsibility for patients and the public to become actively involved in health care provision.
- These changes amount to a significant shift in the relationship between health care provider and recipient; this chapter explores the tensions and opportunities therein.

Public sector workers ... do a fantastic job. They are bound to be the main deliverers of our programmes. But are we going to make patients wait in pain for operations because of some dogma about not using private hospitals, even though they may have spare capacity to do NHS operations? Are we going to force local communities to put up with crumbling Victorian buildings for years and years and years just because we have some ideological objection to a private company building their new hospital?

Tony Blair, 2002

Health services in the UK, as in other developed countries, are going through a period of rapid change. The National Health Service (NHS) constitutes one of the largest organisations to be found in any country. In 2005 it spent £70 billion (2005 prices) and employed over a million people, about 375,000 of whom were nurses.[1] By contrast, the largest private company in Britain, in terms of people employed,

Tesco, came a distant second: it had a turnover in 2005 of £35 billion and employed about 200,000 people. It is therefore unsurprising that attempts to reorganise a huge enterprise such as the NHS have been fraught with difficulty. Many different structures and interest groups are at work, and the 'product' of the organisation – health care – comes in many shapes and sizes. Attempts to fashion new working practices, new funding arrangements and introduce new relationships within the organisation, often by a government operating with short-term political goals, raise, to say the least, complex issues.

In order to provide a workable focus for the chapter, two dimensions of health care organisation will be examined: the changing role of the medical profession and medical practice, and the role of patients and the public in health care. Through examining these two dimensions a number of features of the 'new' NHS should become visible, including changes in the power of the medical profession, the growth of a more plural form of health care delivery and the growth of managed consumerism in health care. What will also become clear is that the organisation of health services in the UK has departed from a centrally organised NHS which is both state funded and state provided. While state funding remains important, local control of finances (through, for example, Foundation Trusts) and a more plural system of providers including those from the private sector, has moved centre stage.

The changing nature of the medical profession and practice

At the time of the General Election in the UK in 2005 the King's Fund (a London-based health policy think-tank) was commissioned by the *Sunday Times* to draw up an 'NHS audit'. This provided an overview of a range of changes in the NHS, and attempted to assess whether their goals had been met. With some provisos the answer was, largely yes. The audit noted that since the turn of the century, the Labour government had committed itself to raising the level of health care expenditure year on year, in order to reach 9 per cent of GDP (around the European average) by 2008. In this the government was on target, as was the case with organisational issues such as reducing waiting times for services, and increasing the numbers of doctors and nurses working in the system. Ten thousand more doctors, 20,000 more nurses and 6500 more therapists were apparently recruited into the service.[2] The audit also found that patient satisfaction with the NHS remained high overall, despite negative media stories. The report suggests that public views of the NHS are therefore influenced less by the media than by actual experience. However, the changes documented by the report only take us so far.

Professional power and managerialism

Useful though such an overview is, in keeping a sense of perspective of developments in the health services, it cannot tell us much about the changing relationships which are accompanying the 'new' Labour agenda. For example, though targets such as shorter waiting times can bring about real benefits to some patients, they may be at the expense of others, whose need may be greater but who do not yet pose a threat to the achievement of the target. Much public discussion and comment has focused on such contradictions and unintended consequences of health care 'modernisation'.[3] In particular, tensions between NHS managers, whose task it is to meet targets, and health care providers who may have other priorities are built into the system. Critics of the 'new' NHS, such as Pollock point to the conflicts that arise under these circumstances. Whereas in the past a 'professional medical ethos' underpinned health care organisation and management, now a more entrepreneurial and 'distinctly "macho" management style' has come to the fore.[4] For Pollock the shift from medical authority and expertise, to management systems based on political decisions and top-down initiatives marks a break with planning to meet need. She argues that this is part of an attempt essentially to privatise the service, an issue to which the chapter returns later.

For the present purposes, it is the question of the changing social relations of health care that are of concern here, and especially the central position of the medical profession. In this respect, changes introduced under the Labour Government's 'modernisation' agenda, have continued those set in train during the Thatcher years. Labour's 'modernising' intentions were set out soon after the 1997 election in *The New NHS: Modern, Dependable*.[5] As we shall see, a raft of initiatives followed this initial statement. Over the years, the changes involved have sought progressively to give more power to managers and reduce the influence of senior doctors on decision making and funding. Thus treasury-driven policies can hope to bypass resistance from the medical profession, and be implemented directly by NHS managers. In the latter half of 2005, for example managers came under intense pressure to reduce costs and stay within their budgets, despite predictions of substantial deficits across the system.[6] As with achieving health service targets in previous years, the failure to meet such goals on the part of managers could lead to the termination of their contracts, a matter far more difficult to achieve if senior hospital consultants were in charge, as previously, of hospital finances.

Having said this, the long-term decline in the influence and power of the medical profession in the health services (and the rise of managerialism) has been much debated. In the 1970s medical sociology was strongly influenced by Eliot Freidson's thesis on the medical profession. This held that in the USA and in other advanced health care systems the medical profession held sway. According to Freidson's approach to the professions it was the degree of autonomy over work practices that provided the basis of medical power. This independence from scrutiny or regulation was then used and extended beyond the borders of medical practice. In so far as the medical profession made *claims* to have jurisdiction over wide areas of life (what to call illness and why, for example) and over the forms and delivery of medical treatment, they were acting, according to Freidson, essentially on a moral terrain. That is, health, illness and health care were seen as issues being decided by the medical profession alone, divorced from lay perspectives.[7] But for Freidson, the medical profession had no more right to decide on health-related issues than any other group in society. Medical knowledge and technical expertise should not, in this view, be used to underpin medical dominance over all matters to do with health and society. The special claims of the professional to have privileged status over health and health care were seen to be illegitimate, and in need of challenge by the wider society.

In an afterword to the second edition of *Profession of Medicine* Freidson noted changes in health care organisation that had occurred since his first edition, which, he said covered the 'Golden Age' of medicine between 1945 and 1965.[8] In particular, the rise of Medicare and Medicaid in the USA, which provided state involvement in 'paying the bills of the elderly and the poor', and of 'large corporate employers' paying for medical insurance, moved the centre of gravity away from the medical profession. Even so, Freidson maintained that 'the loss of extensive political influence and economic independence does not represent the loss of professionalism as I have described it'.[9] While the loss of 'clinical freedom' was 'virtually complete', Freidson could see that all kinds of informal moves by the profession to evade constraints and maintain a high degree of control were always possible. One thinks today, of doctors in the UK context, despite the growth in the power of managers, working their way round waiting-time targets and trying to assert 'clinical judgement' against 'political interference'. To the extent that such actions are successful, the loss of power by the medical profession may be more apparent than real. Freidson saw such power as being differentiated throughout the profession, and exercised in everyday practices, not simply being held or lost by a national unitary body.

Corporatisation and globalisation in health care

There are other factors which point to a more radical shift in the role of the medical profession in the health services. Partly in debate with Freidson, McKinlay and Marceau[10] for example, have argued that the external context of medical practice (in the US context, though much of what they say is applicable increasingly to the UK) marks a major break with the past. Most notably, they argue that 'medical dominance' has given way to 'corporate dominance'. Where once fee-for-service held sway in the US system, 'increasingly concentrated and globalized financial and industrial interests' dominate.[11] These interests not only influence the financing of health care but the way health care organisations are run and medicine practised. Such practice takes on an increasingly 'assembly line' character with the timing, type and tempo of practice being monitored and regulated. Achieving targets in the 'new' NHS are in many respects similar matters of volume and throughput of activity characterised by such specifications.

McKinlay and Marceau make two other points that are relevant to the discussion here. One of these concerns an additional feature of the 'external' environment: the increasingly globalized character of health care. In the USA and in the UK the movement of medical personnel across national boundaries is becoming increasingly common. The European Union, for example, is providing increasing opportunities for mobility for doctors between countries, subject to local licensing and training requirements. At the time of writing, for example, press reports have been appearing of GPs flying into the UK to provide week-end cover from different parts of Europe,[12] and there are now several hundred registered doctors in the UK from France, Germany and Italy alone. Clearly such movements will tend to undermine the position of national professional bodies such as the British Medical Association, as individual doctors operate outside of their influence or control.

Additionally, globalisation also means that health care corporations can operate on an increasingly international basis. Pollock makes the point that private health care companies are looking to increase their penetration into socialised health care systems such as exist in Europe. Pollock argues that a series of meetings of the World Trade Organisation and the General Agreement on Trade in Services in the 1990s paved the way for expanding the range of services being put forward for private investment and competition.[13] Health care is one such service. Debates about the role of US companies such as the United Health Care group, and their attempts to offer packages of care for the chronically ill to the NHS through a scheme called 'Evercare' is only one example of a growing international trend in health care organisation which can be seen to bypass medical jurisdiction.[14, 15]

The second point made by McKinlay and Marceau concerns the increasing competition among health care workers. The rise of what in the USA are often called 'non-physician clinicians' (NPCs) – ranging from nurses, through chiropractors and herbalists to optometrists and podiatrists[16] – constitutes a major challenge to medical dominance. Even though the 'overall pie' of health care, as these authors put it, is likely to increase, so too is the competition between doctors and NPCs. Cooper and Stoflet[17] make the point that the rapid rise in NPCs raises critical issues concerning the quality of care. Of importance here, however, it their observation that the best results from NPC care tend to be at the less complex end of health care, and when such workers are under the direction of a medical physician. In other words although NPCs are on the rise (nurses' sphere of practice in particular is expanding rapidly), they may be operating in such a way as to offer limited challenges to medical dominance. Although a much more pluralistic health care system is likely to develop in countries such as the UK, as it has in the USA, whether this constitutes a major plank in the reduction in the power of medicine, as McKinlay and Marceau seem to think, is open to debate.

From the foregoing discussion it is possible to see important processes at work in the 'new' forms of health care organisation appearing in countries such as the UK and USA. Most importantly, perhaps, the role of the medical profession is being transformed by the rise in bureaucratic and corporate pressures. While the US system has moved to more 'managed' forms of care, socialised systems such as the UK NHS are moving towards greater pluralism, in which private health care delivery will be increasingly evident. It is important, however, not to see a simple process of convergence happening here. Despite changes in medical practice in the USA, writers such as Wholey and Burns[18] argue that this does not constitute moves towards the socialization of health care as a whole, if only because such managed care is not offered to uninsured populations. Similarly, though changes in health care organisation in the UK (more aggressive management, stricter financial control and target setting) offer major challenges to the former dominant position of the medical profession, the NHS remains a centrally funded system of care, with doctors still occupying a key role in the delivery of that care, in what Salter[19] refers to as the 'disposal of resources'. Nonetheless, changes in both systems are marked by a significant shift in the role of the medical profession towards less clinical freedom and a reduction in power.

Before the chapter turns to related and perhaps contrasting changes occurring in the patient's role there are two other aspects of the context of medical organisation and practice that need briefly to be considered. Both are arguably central to understanding the pattern of health care organisation in the current period.

Litigation and health care

The first of these is the change in the legal context of medical practice. It is clear that the protected status of medical practice, enjoyed within socialised systems such as the UK NHS, has reinforced the autonomy and authority of the medical profession. While mistakes and errors may well have occurred in the past, these were seen largely as 'internal' matters. The public either accepted the situation or more cynically saw medicine as a 'closed shop' in which the members – doctors – would protect each other. Unlike the USA, litigation was rare in the UK, and the courts, let alone the police, were not likely to spend much time on medical matters.

During the 1980s and 1990s claims for medical negligence began to spiral. A recent report states that in one English region alone 'clinical negligence claims increased by 72 per cent between 1990 and 1998'.[20] The report goes on to say that nationally claims had doubled from £1.3billion in 1996–7 to £2.6billion in 1999–2000. These trends are a sign, the report says, of an 'increased litigiousness on the part of patients'. Individual claims for conditions such as cerebral palsy, as the result of mistakes occurring at birth or shortly afterwards, can amount to millions of pounds. The risk of having to pay such sums from health service budgets has to be anticipated in financial planning within local health care organisations.

More important, perhaps, from a sociological viewpoint, is what this tells us about the changing nature of health care, and especially the position of doctors within the system. Having enjoyed special privileges the profession is at the time of writing exposed to potential criticism and censure on a regular basis. There is an added level of complexity as a result: the implications for medical care are not always those anticipated by the litigant. In 2005, for example, a leading paediatrician in Britain, Sir Roy Meadow was struck off the medical register by the General Medical Council (GMC) which regulates medical practice in the UK. This followed the case of Sally Clark who had been convicted of the murder of her two sons. Mrs Clark's conviction was overturned in 2003 after a second appeal. The GMC ruled that Meadow's evidence in Mrs Clark's trial (including statistical estimates of the probability that both children had suffered natural deaths) amounted to serious professional misconduct. The chairwoman of the GMC hearing told Meadow that his conduct had 'undermined public confidence in doctors who play a pivotal role in the criminal justice system'.[21] While Mrs Clark welcomed the verdict, Alan Craft, president of the Royal College of Paediatrics argued that 'there will be a huge knock on effect on expert witnesses, both in child protection … and right across the whole field of medicine'. A reduction in the privileged position of the medical profession may make them more accountable. But it may also have the unintended consequence of damaging positive aspects of the wider role that medical practitioners have carried out in the past, with widespread withdrawal from high risk-specialties.[22]

Regulation and accountability in the NHS

The second aspect of the organisation and practice in health care which needs to be noted here concerns increasing regulation and monitoring, alongside accountability through litigation. The influence of scandal on health services is not confined to expert opinion offered in criminal trials. Britain has witnessed a stream of events in the last ten years or more which have led to increasing regulation. Two very different cases stand out. The first is the events surrounding a paediatric unit at Bristol Royal Infirmary in the 1980s where 29 deaths among children undergoing heart surgery were investigated. As a result, two doctors were struck off the medical register and an enquiry lasting three years costing a reported £14m, involving 577 witnesses and over 900,000 documents made a host of recommendations and criticisms.[23] Secrecy and arrogance among doctors were particularly highlighted. The chairman of the enquiry, Sir Ian Kennedy, went on to set up and then chair the Healthcare Commission, whose role it is to 'assess the performance of healthcare organisations, [and] award annual performance ratings' on behalf of the DoH.[24]

The other case which has received enormous professional, policy and public attention concerns the conduct of Dr Harold Shipman, a general practitioner in Manchester, who was found guilty in July 2000 of murdering 15 of his elderly patients, but who probably killed over 200. After his conviction, enquiries were held into the circumstances surrounding his actions, and recommendations were made for future medical practice (Shipman committed suicide in prison in January 2004). In response to this case, and other enquires into medical practice at the time, the Chief Medical Officer, Sir Liam Donaldson, received a report from the GMC on new procedures for 'clinical performance and medical regulation'.[25] Among a range of measures aimed at increasing public confidence in medical practice, the GMC stated that one of its main challenges was to 'ensure the maintenance of national standards and principles of good practice at local level through effective appraisal and clinical governance mechanisms'. Here, again, the autonomy of medical practitioners is being circumscribed by new organisational forms which aim explicitly to limit the ability of doctors to practice without formal oversight or accountability.

Linked to this process is the last aspect of the changing role of medical practice to be discussed here, namely the advent of 'evidence-based health care'. Part of the 'clinical governance' process is the setting of standards and the use of research evidence in the delivery of care. Both of these processes mark a departure from the idea that the individual practitioner should be allowed, indeed encouraged, to use 'clinical judgement' based on initial training and accumulated experience. *National Service Frameworks* now set out to specify the content and form of care for a given area (cancer care, older people, mental health) which aim to increase the quality of care and reduce variation. These frameworks are drawn up by 'external reference groups' comprising professionals, patients, managers and others. Under the auspices of the DoH these reference groups then manage the process of implementation. The DoH sees such developments as a key feature of its 'modernisation' agenda, set in motion in the NHS Plan.[26]

From the more academic direction 'evidence-based health care' (EBHC) seeks to bring the research evidence to bear on treatment decisions. Advocates of this approach such as Sackett et al. have argued that variations in treatment and the need to keep abreast of recent advances in research means that doctors who employ 'selective, efficient patient driven searching, appraisal, and incorporation of the best available evidence can practice evidence based medicine'.[27] In this way these authors hope that EBHC will not be seen simply as an 'ivory tower' initiative. Armstrong[28] has pointed out that, in fact, EBHC can be seen not so much as an 'ivory tower' activity, but rather a move by professional elites to demonstrate to governments their willingness to undertake internal regulation of their activities and embrace clinical governance more fully; embracing a form of 'scientific-bureaucratic' medicine.[29] In this way, as with the GMC's recommendations, more severe regulation of practice and managerial control imposed from 'above' may be minimised.

Of course, as argued earlier, changes in the organisation of care and medical practice do not mean that the position of doctors has lost all continuity with the past. As Hunter[30] has pointed out doctors retain a high degree of social standing. In seeking help for pain and distress it is understandable that despite a loss in public confidence in the medical profession the authority of individual doctors remains high. It also has to be noted that despite much discussion of the loss of faith in the 'grand narrative' of science, medical knowledge and technology retains a legitimacy that outweighs intermittent crises. If this were not the case, patients would not be presenting themselves for medical treatment in record numbers. The demand for medical care shows no sign of abatement. Thus organisational change and political agendas may have profound effects on health care systems, but continuity as well as discontinuity needs to be recognised.

The changing position of the patient in health care organisation

The chapter now alters its angle of perception in order to examine contemporary health care organisation from the patient vantage point. Against the background of what has been said so far a number of key issues immediately come into view. These include: ideas currently being developed to base health care organisation round the 'needs of the patient'; the role of the patient *as* a patient and as a consumer in a system which increasingly emphasises choice; the nature of 'partnership' in health care and specifically in decision making about treatment; initiatives to support self-care and especially the 'Expert Patients Programme' in which responsibility for improvements in care shifts from professional providers to patients themselves. Each of these topics will be looked at in turn.

A patient-led NHS?

In a paper published in the *British Medical Journal* in 1998, Rogers et al. argue that 'the model of health care in which knowledgeable and skilful doctors make decisions on behalf of patients is being increasingly criticised, and more patient centred models of care in which patients play an important role in decisions about their treatment are becoming the norm'.[31] Such new models of health care, these authors argue, should be based on the actions already being taken by lay people in the community. Self-care, the processing of appropriate and culturally sensitive information, and decisions about seeking professional help should all, they argue, be the bedrock of the health care system. In this way 'encouraging demand' for some forms of professional health care can be balanced with 'promoting self-care for other problems'.[32] The overall effect would be to deal with growing demand in the NHS with a form of 'graduated access' where alternative sources of help (self-help groups, help lines and so on) would link informal systems with more formal ones. This graduated approach would restructure health care organisation in ways 'that are sensitive to people's needs and acknowledge that people's use of services is shaped over time'.[33]

In the years that followed, a range of ideas concerning the role of the patient in the health care system in the UK emerged. By 2005, Sir Nigel Crisp, the then Chief Executive of the NHS, was able to argue that having built up the capacity of the NHS, together with improved access and clinical governance to improve quality, a 'more profound change' was appearing on the agenda. Now, Crisp stated, it was necessary 'to change the whole system so that there is more choice, more personalised care, real empowerment of people to improve their health – a fundamental change in our relationships with patients and the public. In other words, to move from a service that does things *to* and *for* its patients to one which is patient led, where the service works *with* patients to support them with their health needs'.[34]

Quoting developments such as the NHS Live programme (local initiatives aimed at involving patients and public in improving services) and the *NHS Improvement Plan*[35] which sets out the terms of change in an NHS being 'patient led', Crisp argued that despite some difficulties the 'direction of travel' is clear. All organisations will need to develop new service models, building on 'current experience and innovation' in which patients are given more choice and control 'wherever possible'. This would result in offering integrated emergency and specialist care to a 'safe, high-quality' standard, and ensuring that all services contribute to 'health promotion, protection and improvement'.[36]

This somewhat heady vision is, at the time of writing, part and parcel of the UK government's 'modernisation' agenda. However rhetorical some aspects of this vision may appear, it clearly marks a departure from earlier forms of official thinking. This is evident in bodies such as the Healthcare Commission, mentioned earlier, where the performance ratings of health care organisations in the future will be based on patients' experiences as well as on objective criteria of quality. In a new system being planned, called the 'Annual Health Check', the Commission 'will for the first time offer patient and public representatives a formal role in judging the quality of services'.[37] In conjunction with the Commission for Patient and Public Involvement in Health, the Healthcare Commission is aiming to involve wider community participation in judging the quality of health care. Despite press reports of serious difficulties with 'Health Forums' that are supposed to help to scrutinise services and influence policy and practice at a local level[38] the process of trying to involve patients in a different role in health care organisation continues.

The idea of a patient-led NHS has an attractive and populist ring to it. In many respects, putting patients' needs in the driving seat and building services round the patient seems logical. Who else's interests should be dominant? The old approach in which 'doctor knows best' and health care is organised for the convenience of the professional is consigned to history, at least in official health policy circles. As Coulter has argued, 'patients have grown up and there is no going back'.[39] Paternalistic health care gives way to a patient-based system, at least as long as patients do not make demands for forms of health care that go completely against accepted medical opinion.

As I have pointed out elsewhere[40] a patient-oriented system of health care does not, of course, guarantee a reduction in problems between providers and consumers. It may have quite the opposite effect. The stress on 'the patient's view' and, where necessary, on patients being encouraged to complain and hold doctors to account may exacerbate forms of 'contestable culture' to be found in late modern societies. Conflict rather than cooperation may result. There have been several examples of this in recent years in the UK's NHS. Mention has already been made of the difficulties surrounding child protection and the role of paediatricians being expert witnesses in court cases. In such circumstances the open criticism of medical expertise may have consequences that go far beyond the immediate cases in hand. While the lay people involved are likely to feel vindicated, the medical profession may feel confused and betrayed by its own professional bodies. Far from producing a new form of cooperation between patients and doctors, resentment and low morale may become widespread.

Added to this are cases in which conflict arises as to the most appropriate form of treatment. If patients are to be given more choice and control 'wherever possible', who is to decide when this point is reached? In the well-documented case of the combined vaccine for measles, mumps and rubella – MMR – medical opinion first raised the possibility of serious side effects in the form of gastrointestinal dis-ease and even autism, and then entered into public dispute as parents began to demand separate vaccination for the three diseases. The Chief Medical Officer, a strong advocate of a patient-led NHS then found himself marshalling all the forces he could to overcome the demand for separate vaccines. In this case medical opinion was split (though the majority view which prevailed was in favour of the combined vaccine) and the patient's view was shown to be mistaken. As Richard Smith, Editor of the *British Medical Journal* at the time stated, although the DoH and government had been stressing choice and the patient view, this could not encompass patients making 'wrong' or 'foolish' decisions, even if telling parents this in the clinic would be difficult.[41] Although the government envisages a new form of health care organisation in which patients are in the driving seat, the much vaunted 'direction of travel' has many humps and traffic jams to deal with.

Consumerism and choice in health care

This brings us to the related question of consumerism and choice, again two central mantras in the 'new' NHS. There is, of course, always a political dimension to health care policies and thus to health care organisation. The emphasis of choice to be found in documents such as Sir Nigel Crisp's *Creating a Patient Led NHS*,[42] is bound up with attempts to decentralise the NHS and create a market type approach. NHS trusts (hospitals, community services) from this viewpoint will become providers competing with each other for health care 'business'. Foundation trusts 'will become "public benefit corporations" to be run as non-profit but nonetheless commercial concerns'.[43] Independent of central government control they will then be free to borrow money on the open market, determine their own priorities and enter into contracts with the private health care sector. Primary Care Trusts will cease almost entirely in providing care directly and will instead commission services from both public and private sectors. Although Pollock argues that patient need will give way to health care based on economic considerations of effectiveness and efficiency,[44] the aim is to create an atmosphere in which patient preferences and demands act as market forces in shaping provision. Though Pollock may be right that wider planning (she gives the example of neonatal care planning in London) becomes more difficult under such circumstances, she may underestimate the level of activity that may be generated around 'unglamorous, complex, costly kinds of care'. This chapter has already mentioned schemes such as Evercare, which aim to sell care packages for those with long-term conditions into the NHS. The 'marketisation' of health care within the NHS (where no fees for treatment to patients will be charged) can extend across the whole range of health care provision.

The changing role of the patient can be seen to help underpin and deliver these new forms of health care within a 'new' NHS. The idea of the informed consumer in health care chimes in with ideas of the 'patient view' and a 'patient-led' service. In fact, as Calnan and Gabe have shown, a market approach to health care in which the patient is seen as a consumer dates from the period in the late 1980s, under a Conservative government, in which hospitals and community units could become Trusts was first mooted. At that time, too, general practitioners in primary care were turned into 'fundholders' and began commissioning services. As these authors state, this altered 'the culture of the NHS from one determined by the preferences and decisions of professionals to one shaped by the views and wishes of its users'.[45]

In such circumstances the GP would act as a proxy for patients, channelling their choices upwards through the system, advocating but not controlling.

Calnan and Gabe go on to note that those general practices that opted to become fundholders delivered shorter waiting times, quicker test results and a more responsive service than those that did not become fundholders.[46] At the same time, Calnan and Gabe also argue that the setting up of Trusts could also reduce choice if this meant that provision in a given area ceased as the result of a loss of a contract through competition. In any event, changes throughout the 1990s, including the *Patient's Charter*[47] led to a rise in dissatisfaction with the NHS, and a rise in complaints. Paradoxically, policies aimed to give patients more of a say in health care can lead to a decline in satisfaction rather than an increase. Whether this is productive of improvements in care is difficult to say. Calnan and Gabe argue that it may be the case that these forms of consumerism in health care actually strengthen the position of managers and politicians in the NHS as they increasingly act 'on behalf of the patient' – just as doctors have claimed in the past.

The current choice agenda constitutes a strong political plank of health policy. It marks a shift from a 'Fordist' emphasis on the production and regulation of health care to a 'Post-Fordist' emphasis on consumption.[48,49] In a series of papers and policy pronouncements since the turn of the century, choice has become the keyword in health care thinking. For example, in December 2003 a strategy paper, *Building on the Best: Choice Responsiveness and Equity in the NHS*, set out a series of proposals concerning choice that played to a strongly populist agenda. Choice, the document argued, was not simply a province of the 'affluent middle classes' but something that all of us want. From 2004, the document stated, patients would be able 'to begin recording their own information securely on the Internet in their own Health Space. In time this will link to their electronic medical record so they can make their preferences known to the clinical team'.[50] Moreover, a wider range of primary care services, easier repeat prescriptions, a choice of hospitals especially if waiting time for surgery extends beyond six months, and greater choice in maternity care and in care at the end of life are all offered. The right information to inform these choices will be 'kitemarked' so that patients will know what they can rely on.

Further papers on 'guiding choice at six months' and information for service providers followed this strategy announcement. In 2004 a document entitled *The NHS Improvement Plan: Putting People at the Heart of Public Services*[51] pulled together a number of these threads in a form that set out clearly the implications of choice and consumerism for health care organisation in the future. In an introduction, the Prime Minister, Tony Blair, stated that 'Our aim is to reshape the NHS, building on the *NHS Plan*[52] so it is not just a national health service but also a personal health service for every patient. We want to provide more choice for every patient, irrespective of the money in their pocket ...'.[53] The *Improvement Plan* went on to state that by the year 2007-8 NHS spending would rise to £90 billion per year, and a raft of measures would be put in place to improve patient choice. These reiterated many of those from previous documents, such as *Building on the Best* and added others concerning long-term care. Patients, the *Plan* states, will be able to choose between a range of providers, and will 'be able to be treated at any facility that meets NHS standards, within the maximum price that the NHS pays for the treatment they need'.[54] In this way choice is linked directly to the development of private as well as public provision within the NHS. It is clear that whatever the limits of consumerism in health care (unlike a CD player or motor car one cannot take a surgical operation 'back to the shop') the idea of state provision and professional control over health care has been abandoned in favour of a mixed economy of care (though still within a tax-based National Health Service) in which patients will increasingly be expected to be active consumers. The most recent development – 'choose and book' – where patients can choose between four hospitals when referred for treatment, only serves to underline the point.

From consumerism to partnership?

One thing leads to another. Even though the future of health care organisation in the UK (and, as has been indicated, it is not alone in pursuing these ideas) seems to be focusing on choice, consumerism, and the 'patient viewpoint', another element is running parallel to those discussed so far. This concerns the idea of 'partnership'. As many governments have found, an over-emphasis on patients rights and prefer-ences carries the risk of alienating professionals and over-stating how far patients are in a position to choose their health care.[55] In both situations serious limitations arise. For example, if a patient is offered the choice of hospitals by a GP, unless that patient is particularly well informed, and has a great deal of information about their respective performance, it is very likely that the question will bounce back – 'What hospital would you go to doctor?' Indeed patients may express the preference for good quality local services, rather than choice as envisaged in government rhetoric.[56] When it comes to decisions about treatment once a service is accessed, again, patients may wish to be involved but find it difficult to balance the risks and benefits of treatment options. In such circumstances 'paternalistic' medical advice may be valued.

In dealing with the reactions of professionals to the emphasis on a 'patient-led' NHS, and the ambiguities of transferring responsibility for choice to the patient, ideas such as partnership have come to the fore. This appears to be less threatening to professionals and somewhat less unrealistic to patients. A recent *Lancet* editorial expresses the professional stance when it states that the government view is that 'the NHS should be patient-led, patients need to complain more, people should have choice and control over the care they get. And doctors are obstacles to this patient–friendly agenda'. Rather, the editorial opines, there is a 'need to strengthen the patient–doctor partnership'.[57] Note the ordering of words here. In previous decades it is likely that sentiments such as this would have been expressed in terms of the 'doctor–patient relationship', a phrase regularly used by the medical profes-sion to explain its position on one or other health care issue. In this way actions could be justified in terms of the patient interest rather than the self-interest of the medical profession. By embracing partnership (and by reversing 'doctor–patient' to 'patient–doctor') the profession signals its intention to try to meet the government half way. Indeed, the term 'partnership' is one much favoured by contemporary governments. It seeks to legitimise a range of activities, from collaboration between private and public sectors in the financing and construction of public services (including building hospitals, schools and prisons) to various initiatives at com-munity level, including tackling crime and anti-social behaviour. In these areas of public policy the emphasis is on 'shared information, shared evaluations and shared responsibility'.[58]

In the health care sector 'partnership' has come to take on several meanings. As Coulter has pointed out, the idea of partnership in health goes beyond public representatives serving on health policy committees, or even serving as lay members on health care bodies, such as Trusts. In such circumstances, patient involvement may amount to little more than unrepresentative individuals serving on bodies where other 'stakeholders' and political priorities (such as meeting government targets) hold sway. For Coulter, the idea of partnership goes much further; to the heart of the 'one-to-one clinical encounter'. This means that partnership should cover 'shared decision-making, including patients' information needs, the evaluation and use of patient decision aids, and strategies for training health professionals to elicit patients' values and preferences and engage them in decisions about their care'.[59] Citing a wide body of research and a special issue of the *British Medical Journal*[60] given over to the topic, Coulter asks, 'is shared decision-making doomed to remain the obsession of a few academic pointy heads?' and 'what can be done to move it into the mainstream?'

Three years later, in a further discussion of the topic Coulter sounded even less sure that shared decision making would prove to be the hallmark of partnership in health care in the future.[61] Again, citing a wide body of literature, together with a series of new studies, Coulter argues that a full picture of partnership displays many different features. As with choice, it seems clear that patients' views may not always coincide with the dominant ideas of policy makers, or, indeed, those of 'pointy head' academics. Although some of the latter argue that professionals should always seek to help 'patients to make informed medical decisions for themselves'.[62] Coulter notes that research also indicates that some patients prefer to remain uninformed and to delegate shared decision making responsibility to the doctor. Coulter goes on to outline a series of debating points about partnership and shared decision making, including findings that indicate that patients wish to know doctors' opinions as well as wanting 'objective information'. She also refers to research that questions assumptions governing the widespread adoption of decision aids.

Whatever the difficulties facing the implementation of shared decision making as part of a partnership approach to health care organisation, it is clear that it will remain a key feature of government policy. As Gabe et al. have pointed out, 'partnership has superseded an earlier model of patient involvement based on consumerism, patients' charters and the need for the health service to be responsive to knowledgeable individuals who shop round for their health care'.[63] Citing the influential work of Charles and her colleagues,[64,65] Gabe et al. argue that shared decision making and the exchange of information between patients and doctors may take different forms as an illness trajectory unfolds. Thus in the early stages, when diagnosis and tests need to be undertaken a range of expert opinion may come into play and be the dominant voice. During a period of reflection and decision making about treatment options a more 'shared' approach may be feasible, though time and other constraints play a part here. Following treatment, and hopefully during recovery, the emphasis may shift once again towards the patient, with the professional supporting self care and rehabilitation. Gabe et al. also query that even in this more developed approach it may be that patients are not 'ready or willing to take on increased decision-making responsibilities'.[66]

One of the difficulties in fashioning partnership and shared decision making strategies is that health care covers a very wide range of health related experiences, with patients and health care professionals bringing many different factors into a given encounter. In health care one size cannot fit all. Gabe et al. raise a crucial factor in this context, namely age. In the case of paediatric care, for example, the question of the legal and social status of the child (or young person) in the health care system introduces a particular dynamic into proceedings. In these circumstances it is rarely the case that 'the patient' appears alone in the clinical encounter, and equally rare that decisions about treatment will be made by the young person without the influence of a parent. Indeed, for infants and very young children such parental involvement may be the only way to make relevant decisions. While there is emphasis today on 'children's rights' in health care (as in other areas of life) Gabe et al. argue that this complicates as much as clarifies the situation. Both national and international policies concerning children in health care stress *both* the need for professionals to act to protect the child and for the 'child's voice to be heard'.[67] These two strictures may cut across each other in given situations, for example in undertaking invasive life saving treatment, or judging that the child's preferences will lead to a 'failure to protect'.

Children are not alone in posing a major challenge to the development of patient partnership. Older patients, especially those whose cognitive abilities are impaired, or who are being cared for a by a close relative or friend may not be (or wish to be) the sole decision maker interacting with the professional. Indeed, many if not most patients are likely to be embedded in a network of more or less supportive relationships. In some cultural settings it may be quite unrealistic to think of patients as individual actors, equivalent, on the other side of the table, to the autonomous professional. The clinical encounter, in this sense at least, is not a meeting of equals. For patients, encounters with doctors will be surrounded by a range of emotional and social factors all bearing on the agenda they bring to the 'partnership' process. For doctors, bureaucratic, legal and professional factors provide guidelines for approaching each 'case' in turn. While some aspects of the encounter can therefore be regarded as open to the development of partnership and perhaps shared decision making, this is unlikely ever to characterise the encounter as a whole. Their respective roles and 'assumptive worlds' are too distinct.

One other aspect of partnership is worth noting at this point. A great deal of medical activity in health care organisations deals with the prescribing of drugs. Here, too, the government has proposed changes in the patient's role and thus in the organisation of health care. In 2003, as part of the government £30m 'Pharmacy in the Future' programme, a new body entitled 'Medicines Partnership' set out a series of new steps to modernise public health pharmacy and outline new roles for both professionals (including nurses and community pharmacists) and patients alike. In this new vision, the earlier emphasis on encouraging patient compliance, in which patients were expected to follow 'doctor's orders' is supplanted by the notion of concordance. This new approach emphasises the idea that prescriber and consumer should enter into a shared decision-making process and arrive at a mutually agreed approach to the prescribing and taking of medicines. The resulting 'concordance' between patient and prescriber should overcome, it is hoped, the faults of compliance where patients' views remained unexamined in the prescribing process. Non-compliance, and the waste of drugs never taken, should both be addressed by this route. The Medicines Partnership states that 'the initiative is aimed at helping patients to get the most out of medication by involving them as partners in prescribing decisions and supporting them in medicine taking'.[68] A task force has been set up to implement concordance and partnership in medicine taking throughout the NHS.

As elsewhere on this new health care terrain, questions about concordance have been quick to emerge. Britten for example has argued that assumptions about changes in patient behaviour and their implications in clinical encounters need to be tested against first-hand observational research. In fact, she states, where such research has been carefully conducted it indicates that the expression of patient preferences may lead to the issuing of prescriptions that are not clinically needed. In one study, when asked why they had done so, doctors stated that it had occurred 'in order to maintain relationships with patients'.[69] This suggests that some patients may be pressurising their doctors to take decisions against their clinical judgement. It appears that patients' priorities may therefore be very different from prescribers' priorities or indeed from the priorities that the prescribers presume their patients to have'.[70] The agendas, again, of both 'partners' may simply be too different for 'concordance' to be arrived at with any ease. Patients may be more concerned with the demands of their social situation and 'moral concerns' (that is, with not taking drugs unnecessarily and appearing not to be seen as dependent on medication)[71] than worrying too much about the fine detail of medicine taking itself. Britten states that 'clinicians who are trying to give their patients the best evidence about treatment options and to present balanced information about risks and benefits may find it difficult to take this on board'.[72] As with shared decision making more generally, pursuing concordance may alter some aspects of health care delivery, but the jury must be out as to how meaningful this may become as a part of new organisational structure.

Self-care and the expert patient

This brings us to the final stage in plans for changes in the role of the patient in the new NHS – that of self-care and the 'expert patient'. Mention has already been made of the NHS Improvement Plan,[73] in which the government has set out its proposals for reshaping the NHS. A central chapter in this plan, Chapter 3, deals with 'Supporting People with Long-term Conditions to Live Healthy Lives'. The chapter states that 'about 60 per cent of adults report some form of long-term or chronic health problem'.[74] As a result, the use of health care increases with the number of problems reported ('the 15 per cent of people with three or more problems account for almost 30 per cent of inpatient days'). Although it is not clear how the 60 per cent figure has been arrived at and what range of problems it is referring to, the Improvement Plan goes on to describe a set of arrangements that will meet the challenge of chronic illness in the community. At the more severe end of the spectrum, those with 'highly complex conditions' will be offered 'case management'. This will involve the advent of over 3000 'community matrons' by 2008, who will 'co-ordinate the contribution of all the different professionals who can help, anticipate and deal with problems before they lead to worsening health or hospitalisation'.[75] Since the publication of the plan, two reports have cast doubt on the effectiveness of this approach,[76, 77] but it is still being pursued.

At the intermediate level, 'higher-risk' patients with serious chronic disease that is not 'complex' in character (such as asthma, diabetes or depression) will receive 'disease management', largely within the primary care setting. In heart disease, for example, measures such as checking blood pressure or cholesterol levels and ensuring that support is given for stopping smoking will be offered. The development of *National Service Frameworks*, together with guidance from the National Institute of

Health and Clinical Excellence will help to underpin this kind of approach. 'Strong financial incentives' under the new GP contract, it is hoped, will help doctors 'seek out patients who can benefit from this kind of support and demonstrate that they are making a real difference to their health'.[78]

However, it is at the third level, affecting 70–80 per cent of patients, that 'self-management' is seen as the cornerstone of the Improvement Plan. This combines the idea of self-care in 'population-wide prevention', and self-management with respect to the bulk of existing chronic conditions. In the case of prevention, self-care shades across into the well-worn paths of stressing the individual's responsibility for maintaining their health. But it is the area of chronic illness that newer and more innovative forms of health care are proposed. Central to this, and drawing on 'international experience', the Plan states, is the 'Expert Patients Programme' (EPP). In this programme, 'using trained non-medical leaders as educators, people with arthritis and other long-term conditions have been equipped with the skills to manage their own conditions'. 'By 2008', the Plan states, 'it will have been rolled out throughout the NHS, enabling thousands more patients to take greater control of their own health and their own lives'.[79]

The international experience alluded to in the Plan comes from one particular source: Stanford University in the USA. There, a 'chronic disease self-management programme' (CDSMP) pioneered and led by Kate Lorig[80,81] has trained 'lay tutors', in key self-management skills. These tutors then run courses for other chronically ill patients, without the oversight of medical practitioners. The EPP in Britain (adopted at present only in England with a parallel initiative in Wales) is essentially the CDSMP, with minor changes. The course in question comprises six two-hour weekly sessions, teaching the participants not about their disease (in the British version anyone suffering from a long-term condition can sign up to go on the EPP) but skills in areas such as exercise, fatigue management, communication with professionals, and diet. The underlying theory of the programme, based on the work of the American psychologist, Albert Bandura, is that an increase in the level of 'self-efficacy' will help people feel more in control of their condition and of their lives.

The EPP runs an active website for patients and health care practitioners.[82] Those interested can sign up to a regular 'e-update' on the EPP and find out how to participate, or even become a lay tutor. It is clear from the website, as well as recent media coverage that many patients who have volunteered to go on the course, and who have completed at least most of the six modules, claim to have benefited from the experience. On the EPP website, under a 'views from patients and professionals' heading, 'Cathy', for example, states that as a result of being on the Programme she has been able 'to take some positive steps for the future'. In a poem written by a 'Sue Jump', Sue states that 'So now, I am a tutor helping others to find the pearl'. And despite misgivings about the programme, especially the notion of patients as 'experts' among some sections of the medical profession[83] even some doctors have welcomed the programme. On the EPP website, GP Nicola Jones states that as a result of the Programme 'patients demonstrate resourcefulness, not asking "what should I do?" but rather "do you think this will work". It's about control'.

The problem arises, however, when a wider evaluation of the Programme is attempted. To date there has been limited systematic study of the Programme in the UK, though an evaluation of the Programme's implementation and a randomised controlled trial have been carried out by the National Primary Care Research and Development Centre at Manchester. Their two reviews of the Programme's progress paint a mixed picture, both of the practical problems encountered in setting up the course, recruiting patients and tutors to them, and 'embedding' the Programme fully in the NHS.[84,85] Claims therefore made by the Department of Health that this programme is supported by research evidence need to be treated with caution. Most of the studies of 'self-management' in chronic illness (whether using the kind of approach advocated by Lorig in the USA and the EPP in Britain or not) are of 'condition-specific' programmes, for disorders such as arthritis or asthma. A recent review of this literature, covering three conditions showed some benefits in the short term, in some studies, but little if any long-term effectiveness.[86,87] Lorig's own research on the CDSMP showed some positive outcomes in the short term at six months (though not on all measures, including psychological well-being) but much less in an uncontrolled follow up at 2 years.[88,89] Such findings are, perhaps understandable. If the attraction of being involved in the programme helps overcome participants' previous sense of isolation short-term benefits may be evident. It is quite a different matter to sustain positive changes over a longer time span – essential in the case of chronic conditions. It is highly likely that social factors and the progression of the condition may reassert themselves with the passage of time.

Conclusion

Initiatives such as the EPP hold out the promise of new forms of health care organisation that will be radically different from the past. This chapter has explored changes in both the role of the doctor and of the patient that seem to be emblematic of these proposed changes. What ties them together, perhaps, is the emphasis on the patient's viewpoint, whether we consider reductions in professional power, the growth of regulation or the rise of a 'patient-led' NHS. Taylor and Bury have called this process 'care transition', suggesting a major break with the past.[90] There is much to commend such a refocusing of health care organisation and service delivery to meet new demands. Enough has been said to indicate that a number of agendas are at work here. Health care and health services are at base political issues, and 'new' forms of heath care organisation as described earlier clearly chime in with 'new' Labour's approach to the public sector more generally. Here, private financing, private provision and an emphasis of consumerism are brought to bear on 'monolithic' public services such as the NHS.

The underlying contradiction in such an approach lies in the fact that the emphasis on the patient view or on patient self-care has not emerged directly from patients themselves, but from a centralised 'top-down' set of initiatives and 'reorganisation' coming from government. This is why, when careful research is undertaken, patients do not often or regularly confirm the assumptions held. It is unlikely that they could. The idea of the 'patient viewpoint' is fundamentally problematic, if only because patients are many and various. In addition, there are many areas of health care in which high-quality medical expertise is essential to good outcomes. Shifting the balance of power (to use the title of yet another and earlier government document) towards the patient may be important in offsetting the dysfunctional aspects of a 'paternalistic' form of medicine and too much professional control in shaping health care organisation. But however useful the rhetoric of the 'patient's viewpoint' may be in this process, it is unlikely to alter the experience of the vast majority of practitioners and patients in the health care system as a whole. Whether a more realistic approach to health care organisation can be developed, in which clinical expertise and patients' varying needs can be reconciled more appropriately, only time will tell.

Discussion topics

- Are we witnessing the demise of the medical profession's dominance of health care provision?
- What might be the benefits, disadvantages and responsibilities of becoming an 'expert patient'?
- Can the doctor–patient relationship be transformed into a partnership based on shared decision making? What would the consequences be?

Further reading

Calnan, M. and Gabe, J. (2001) From consumerism to partnership? Britain's national health service at the turn of the century. *International Journal of Health Services*, 31(1): 119–31.

This paper examines the extent of 'medical dominance' and 'consumerism' in today's health care system.

Department of Health (2004) *The NHS Improvement Plan: Putting People at the Heart of Public Services*. Cmnd 6268. London: The Stationery Office.

This policy document sets out the terms of health care 'reform' developed during the Blair years.

Hunter, D. (1994/2005) From tribalism to corporatism: the managerial challenge to medical dominance. In J. Gabe, D. Kelleher and G. Williams (eds), *Challenging Medicine*. London: Routledge.

This chapter examines the rise of managerialism in health care and explores the extent to which it has undermined the autonomy and authority of the medical profession.

Pollock, A.M. (2004) *NHS PLC: The Privatisation of Our Health Care*. London: Verso.

Pollock's book offers a challenging and controversial argument concerning 'privatisation' in the NHS.

References

1   Buchan, J. (2004) International rescue? The dynamics and policy implications of the international recruitment of nurses to the UK. *Health Services Research and Policy*, 9 (Supplement 1): 11.
2   King's Fund (2005) *An Independent Audit of the NHS Under Labour*. London: King's Fund, p. 4.

3   Healthcare Commission (2005) *State of Healthcare 2005*. London: Commission for Healthcare Audit and Inspection.
4   Pollock, A.M. (2004) *NHS PLC: The Privatisation of Our Health Care*. London: Verso, p. 54.
5   Department of Health (1997) *The New NHS: Modern, Dependable*. Cmnd 3807. London: Department of Health.
6   Mooney, H. (2005) Mass redundancies expected as SHAs tackle £750m shortfall. *Health Service Journal*, 13 July.
7   Freidson, E. (1970/1988) *Profession of Medicine: A Study of the Sociology of Applied Knowledge*. Chicago: University of Chicago Press, p. 343.
8   Freidson, E. (1970/1988) ibid., p. 384.
9   Freidson, E. (1970/1988) ibid., p. 385.
10 McKinlay, J.B and Marceau, L.D. (2002) The end of the golden age of doctoring. *International Journal of Health Services*, 32(2): 379–416.
11 McKinlay, J.B. and Marceau, L.D. (2002) ibid., p. 381.
12 BBC, 17 June 2005.
13 Pollock, A.M. (2004) ibid., p. 61.
14 Smith, R. (2003) Improving the management of chronic disease. *BMJ*, 327: 12
15 Mayor, S. (2005) Case management to be used for people with chronic conditions. *BMJ*, 330: 112
16 McKinlay, J.B. and Marceau, L.D. (2002) ibid., pp. 391–2.
17 Cooper, R. and Stoflet, S. (2004) Diversity and consistency: the challenge of maintaining quality in a multidisciplinary workforce. *Journal of Health Services Research and Policy*, 9 (Supplement 1): 39–47.
18 Wholey, D.R. and Burns, I.R (2000) Tides of change: the evolution of managed care in the United States. In C.E. Bird, P. Conrad and A.M. Fremont (eds), *Handbook of Medical Sociology*. Upper Saddle River, NJ: Prentice Hall, pp. 217–37.
19 Salter, B. (2004) *The New Politics of Medicine*. Houndmills: Palgrave Macmillan.
20 National Audit Office (2001) *Handling Clinical Negligence Claims in England*. London: National Audit Office, p. 11.
21 Dyer, C. (2005) Professor Roy Meadow struck off. *BMJ*, 331: 177.
22 *Lancet* (2005) A dismal and dangerous verdict against Roy Meadow. *The Lancet*, 366: 277.
23 Department of Health (2001) *Report of the Public Inquiry into Children's Heart Surgery at the Bristol Royal Infirmary 1984–1985*. Cmnd 5207. London: The Stationery Office.
24 www.healthcarecommission.org.uk
25 GMC (2005) *Developing Medical Regulation: A Vision for the Future*. London: GMC.
26 Department of Health (2000) *The NHS Plan: A Plan for Investment and a Plan for Reform*. Cmnd 4818–1. London: The Stationery Office.
27 Sackett, D.L., Rosenberg, W.M.C., Gray, M.J.A., Haynes, R.B. and Richardson, W.S. (1996) Evidence based medicine: what it is and what it isn't. *British Medical Journal*, 312: 71–2.
28 Armstrong, D. (2002) Clinical autonomy, individual and collective: the problem of changing doctors' behaviour. *Social Science and Medicine*, 55(10): 1771–7.
29 Harrison, S. (2002) New labour, modernisation and the medical labour process. *Journal of Social Policy*, 31(3): 465–85.

30 Hunter, D. (1994/2005) From tribalism to corporatism: the managerial challenge to medical dominance. In J. Gabe, D. Kelleher and G. Williams (eds) *Challenging Medicine*. London: Routledge.
31 Rogers, A., Entwistle, V. and Pencheon, D. (1998) Managing demand: a patient led NHS: managing demand at the interface between lay and primary care. *British Medical Journal*, 316: 1818.
32 Rogers, A., Entwistle, V. and Pencheon, D. (1998) ibid., p. 1816.
33 Rogers, A., Entwistle, V. and Pencheon, D. (1998) ibid., p. 1819.
34 Department of Health (2005) *Creating a Patient-Led NHS: Delivering the NHS Improvement Plan*. London: Department of Health, p. 3.
35 Department of Health (2004) *The NHS Improvement plan: Putting People at the Heart of Public Services*. Cmnd 6268. London: The Stationery Office.
36 Department of Health (2005) ibid., p. 5.
37 www.healthcarecommission.org.uk
38 *Guardian*, 11 May 2005
39 Coulter, A. (1999) Paternalism or partnership? Patients have grown up – and there's no going back. *British Medical Journal*, 319: 719–20.
40 Bury, M. (2005) *Health and Illness*. Cambridge: Polity Press, p. 104.
41 Smith, R. (2002) The discomfort of patient power. *British Medical Journal*, 324: 497–8.
42 Department of Health (2005) ibid.
43 Pollock, A.M. (2004) ibid., p. 71
44 Pollock, A.M. (2004) ibid., p. 72.
45 Calnan, M. and Gabe, J. (2001) From consumerism to partnership? Britain's National Health Service at the turn of the century. *International Journal of Health Services*, 31(1): 120.
46 Calnan, M. and Gabe, J. (2001) ibid., p. 121.
47 Department of Health (1991) *The Patient's Charter*. London: Department of Health.
48 Harrison, S. (2002) New labour, modernisation and the medical labour process. *Journal of Social Policy*, 31(3): 465–85.
49 Pickstone, J.E. (2000) Production, community and consumption: the political economy of twentieth century medicine. In R. Cooter and J.E. Pickstone (eds) *Medicine in the Twentieth Century*. London: Harwood.
50 Department of Health, (2003) *Building on the Best: Choice, Responsiveness and Equity in the NHS*. London: Department of Health, p. 3
51 Department of Health (2004) ibid.
52 Department of Health (2000) ibid.
53 Department of Health (2004) ibid., p. 4.
54 Department of Health (2004) ibid., p. 6.
55 *Lancet* (2005) Will consumerism lead to better health? *The Lancet*, 366: 343.
56 Consumers' Association (2005) Government choosing the wrong choices for healthcare says. *Which?* www.which.net/press//releases/health.
57 *Lancet* (2005) Will consumerism lead to better health? *The Lancet*, 366: 343.
58 Calnan, M. and Gabe, J. (2001) ibid., p. 127.
59 Coulter, A. (2002) Whatever happened to shared decision making? *Health Expectations*, 5: 186.
60 *British Medical Journal* (1999) Special theme issue: embracing patient partnership.
61 Coulter, A. (2005) Shared decision-making: the debate continues. *Health Expectations*, 8: 95–6.

62 Coulter, A. (2005) ibid.
63 Gabe, J., Olumide, G. and Bury, M. (2004) 'It takes three to tango': a framework for understanding patient partnership in paediatric clinics. *Social Science and Medicine*, 59: 1072.
64 Charles, C., Gafni, A. and Whelan, T. (1997) Shared decision-making in the medical encounter: what does it mean? (Or it takes at least two to tango). *Social Science and Medicine*, 44(5): 681–92.
65 Charles, C., Gafni, A. and Whelan, T. (1999) Decision-making in the physician-patient encounter. Revisiting the shared treatment decision-making model. *Social Science and Medicine*, 49: 651–61.
66 Gabe, J., Olumide, G. and Bury, M. (2004) ibid.
67 Gabe, J., Olumide, G. and Bury, M. (2004) ibid., p. 1073.
68 www.medicine-parternership.org
69 Britten, N. (2004) Patients' expectations of consultations. *British Medical Journal*, 328: 416.
70 Britten, N. (2003) Does a prescribed treatment match a patient's priorities? *British Medical Journal*, 327: 840.
71 Horne, R., Weinman, J. and Hankins, M. (1999) The beliefs about medicines questionnaire: the development and evaluation of a new method for assessing the cognitive representation of medication. *Psychology and Health*, 14(1): 1–24.
72 Britten, N. (2003) ibid., p. 840.
73 Department of Health (2004) ibid.
74 Department of Health (2004) ibid., p. 34.
75 Department of Health (2004) ibid., p. 38.
76 Hutt, R., Rosen, R. and McCauley, J. (2004) *Case Managing Long Term Conditions: What Impact Does It Have in the Treatment of Older People?* London: King's Fund.
77 Roland, M., Dusheiko, M., Gravelle, H. and Parker, S. (2005) Follow up of people aged 65 and over with a history of emergency admissions: analysis of routine admission data. *British Medical Journal*, 330: 289–92.
78 Department of Health (2004) ibid., p. 37.
79 Department of Health (2004) ibid., p. 36.
80 Lorig, K., Sobel, D.S., Stewart, A.L., Brown, B.M., Bandura, A., Ritter, P., Gonzalez, V.M., Laurent, D.D. and Holman, H.R. (1999) Evidence suggesting that a chronic disease self-management program can improve health status while reducing hospitalization, a randomized trial. *Medical Care*, 37(1): 5–14.
81 Lorig, K.E., Ritter, P., Stewart, A.L., Sobel, D.S., Brown, B.W., Bandura, A., Gonzalez, V.M., Laurent, D.D. and Holman, H.R. (2001) Chronic disease self-management program, 2-year health status and health care utilization outcomes. *Medical Care*, 39(11): 1217–23.
82 www.expertpatients.nhs.uk
83 Shaw, J. and Baker, M. (2004) 'Expert patient': dream or nightmare? *British Medical Journal*, 328: 723–4.
84 Kennedy, A., Gately, C. and Rogers, A. (2004) *Assessing the Process of Embedding EPP in the NHS: Preliminary Study of PCT Pilot Sites*. Manchester: National Primary Care Research and Development Centre.
85 EPP Evaluation Team (2005) *Process Evaluation of the EPP: Report II*. Manchester: National Primary Care Research and Development Centre, University of Manchester.
86 Newman, S., Steed, L. and Mulligan, K. (2004) Self-management interventions for chronic illness. *Lancet*, 364: 1523–37.

87 Bury, M., Newbould, J. and Taylor, D. (2005) *A rapid review of knowledge regarding lay-led self-management of chronic illness*. London: National Institute for Health and Clinical Excellence.

88 Lorig, K., Sobel, D.S., Stewart, A.L., Brown, B.M., Bandura, A., Ritter, P., Gonzalez, V.M., Laurent, D.D. and Holman, H.R. (1999) ibid.

89 Lorig, K.E., Ritter, P., Stewart, A.L., Sobel, D.S., Brown, B.W., Bandura, A., Gonzalez, V.M., Laurent, D.D. and Holman, H.R. (2001) ibid.

90 Taylor, D. and Bury, M. (2007) Chronic illness, expert patients and care transition. *Sociology of Health and Illness*, 29(1): 27–45.

10

Changing Concepts of International Health

Vanessa Pupavac

- The health policies of western governments are aimed primarily at addressing the health needs of their own populations, but international agencies such as the World Health Organisation, have also been established to tackle health problems globally.
- A central aim of these agencies is to address the pressing health problems of the third world. The policies and priorities developed to achieve this reflect the concerns of the major donor countries.
- In the immediate post-war period international health policy was driven by the imperative of social and economic *modernisation*, and sought to equip the third world with the high technology health care systems found in the West.
- Since then, the modernization agenda has come under sustained criticism, and international health agencies are increasingly adopting less ambitious programmes which emphasise *sustainability*, and the pursuit of 'well-being'.
- The debates behind the changing conception of international health policy are examined here, and the implications for third world development are assessed.

There is no bigger test for humanity than the crisis of global health. Solving it will require the full commitment of our hearts and minds. We need both. Without compassion, we won't do anything. Without science, we can't do anything. So far, we have not applied all we have of either.

Bill Gates, 2005

International health policy in the first two decades after the Second World War was ambitious and linked to the national development of the newly independent states. International support for ambitious health goals reflected Cold War rivalry between the Western and Soviet blocs for political influence in the Third World. Developing countries enjoyed a high degree of legitimacy internationally following successful anti-colonial struggles. The aspirations of developing countries were represented in the Non-Aligned Movement whose voice internationally belied the relative weakness of its members. The elevated status of developing countries within the UN organisations in this period was important for setting the high ambitions of international development and international health.

The World Health Organisation (WHO) was founded in 1948 with a constitution which set out its objective as 'the attainment by all peoples of the highest possible level of health', which it defined as 'a state of complete physical, mental and social well-being and not merely the absence of disease or infirmity'.[1]

The rise and fall of modernization strategy

Western states were ambivalent about the development of non-western states, as potential future rival powers in their own right or as states within the Soviet orbit of influence. But western qualms over international development and power shifting internationally away from North America and Europe were suppressed by consciousness that if the West did not support developing states, they could turn to the Soviet bloc for support. Western policy makers supported western models of modernisation, hoping that the convergence of living standards through industrial development would lead to the convergence of cultural and political values, and realise progress without social instability.[2] Western policy makers hoped too that the adoption of modern urban life styles and the nuclear family would reduce population growth in developing countries. Population growth was a major western preoccupation, informed by security concerns, which equated demography with national power.[3] Accordingly, much western international health funding related to family planning programmes.[4]

International health policy in the political climate of the Cold War was planned on the assumption that non-western states would be industrialised and reach the same levels of development as western industrialised states. The goals of international health policy were nothing less than the eradication of disease and the establishment of modern medicine and modern hospitals with medically trained staff. The motto of international health policy in this period may be summed up as: eradicate and cure.

Eradicate and cure

The Malaria Eradication Programme (MEP), a central plank of the WHO's approach in the 1950s and 1960s, symbolised the high ambitions of international health policy in the first two decades of international development. The high ambitions were informed by great optimism in science and the possibilities of modern medicine. They also involved expectations of equality between countries including expectations that populations in developing countries should enjoy the levels of physical health and absence of disease experienced by populations in developed countries. The MEP gained some early successes in rolling back the spread of malaria, essentially through the use of pesticides to control malaria-carrying mosquitoes, but began to experience difficulties as resistance developed to the pesticides used, including DDT.

If MEP was ultimately unsuccessful, the eradication of smallpox represented an unprecedented international effort to eradicate disease. Eradicating smallpox was technically easier because it was transmitted by human-to-human contact and was not an insect-borne disease. In turn since the interventions required were simpler and effective, countries were enthused at all levels of society to implement the smallpox eradication programme by the speed of results witnessed in the countries initially targeted.

Rising health expectations and development

Health was not simply seen as important in its own right, but as important in promoting development. First, disease eradication was seen as vital to promote a healthier workforce when many workers, or potential workers, were debilitated by malaria and other diseases. Second, disease eradication was seen as important in facilitating development programmes by freeing up land plagued by malaria, sleeping sickness, river blindness and other diseases for cultivation and development. Third, health improvements were seen as promoting new values among populations conducive to development. Repeatedly the international health literature made a link between raising health expectations and raising the horizon of expectations among populations more broadly. Fatalism and risk aversion were seen as major cultural obstacles to development, which health improvements could tackle. From this perspective, health programmes helped foster entrepreneurialism. The economist Wilfred Malenbaum observed that:

Health inputs in physical facilities have a high demonstration effect on the power of man to influence his own destiny. For the bulk of the poor, and especially the poor peasant, the happenings of life tend to be accepted as pre-ordered, however harsh their influence. Health programs may serve to challenge the inevitability of this sequence. Since the consequences of new health facilities are highly visible, the peasant's own decisions on other measures, and especially on his everyday work activities, may begin to alter the formerly pre-ordered prospects.[5]

Health programmes required acceptance by communities to work. A major concern of international policy makers was how to encourage people to follow health programmes. Cultural anthropologists like Margaret Mead were consulted by the WHO. Mead quotes one 1950s' health education initiative, which asked:

How can you influence people living in rural areas to get water from safe sources? How can you overcome the resistance of people to modern medicines? How can we educate the public that sanitary hygiene plays a big part in the prevention of leprosy and other contagious diseases? How can we influence people to change their present unsatisfactory village sites to more healthy ones?[6]

Public compliance with health education lessons could not be treated in isolation from their general expectations. Health messages succeeded where people had raised expectations about their lives. Mead cites Egyptian researchers who observed that:

In many rural areas people lived in an environment offering many hazards and few resources. In their present struggle for existence their greatest need was to be able to look forward to a better level of living. An appeal to them to change their food and health habits generally fell on deaf ears, because they were so well aware of their own insecurities and so used to them that they had in the past made all the adjustments that seemed possible. Hence they appeared uncertain and sceptical about new proposals to alter their way of living. Yet suggestions about new uses of their existing resources, and particularly evidence of some small successes, might make them aware of the possibility of escape from the ceaseless effort to achieve a bare existence.[7]

Initially there were concerns that people would need to be encouraged to use modern medicine, but these concerns were soon superseded by concerns about the overuse of modern hospitals and medicine. Mead's own study is ambivalent about the benefits of modernisation for well-being, as will be discussed later. From the late 1960s the ambitions of international health policy began to be tempered.

Retreat from eradicate and cure

The lesson for international health policy was drawn from the failure of malaria eradication, rather than the successful eradication of smallpox. Certainly malaria eradication presented more difficulties than smallpox eradication and the MEP had run into serious problems over pesticide resistance. However, the MEP was not simply abandoned because of technical difficulties, but the withdrawal of political and financial support from major donor states, notably the United States. The withdrawal of support was related to international political and domestic cultural concerns. Not least the value the MEP placed on DDT and other pesticides to control malaria fell foul of the nascent environmental thinking in the West, encapsulated in Rachel Carson's *Silent Spring*.[8] Carson blamed her own cancer on chemical pesticides and her passionate attack against DDT and other chemical pesticides poisoning the planet gained a wide hearing in western countries.

More broadly the ideas behind the MEP were out of step with the changing international development strategies which were moving away from modernisation towards sustainable development. The shift was led by fears that modernisation strategies were fostering social and political problems. Dudley Seers, director of the influential Institute of Development Studies, University of Sussex, alerted in the late 1960s that 'it looks as if economic growth not merely may fail to solve social and political difficulties; certain types of growth can actually cause them'.[9] Uneven development and sharp inequalities within developing countries questioned modernisation strategies. Fears over existing strategies were brought home to western officials by the experience of political assassinations and civil riots domestically, the Vietnam War and the 1973 Oil Crisis internationally, which rekindled Malthusian fears over resources and suggested that developing countries could hold Western states to ransom over raw materials. Meanwhile Third World nationalism was on the wane and developing countries exercised waning influence on international development strategies including international health policy.

The sustainable development model

The sustainable development model was codified from the 1970s and 1980s in documents such as the Brandt report *North–South: A Programme for Survival*, published in 1980. Sustainable development policy makers challenged the idea that 'the whole world should copy the models of highly industrialized countries'.[10] Industrial development as the goal of international development was replaced by basic needs policies pioneered by bodies such as the International Labour Organization.[11,12,13] Investment in low or medium technology, not industrialisation, and more small-scale rural development projects was considered appropriate for developing countries.[14] The policy implied continued reliance on self-generated income activities and subsistence farming for the vast majority of developing countries' populations.

The changing international development strategies revised international health policy goals from the ambitious disease eradication and cure model to a more modest disease management and prevention model and from modern high-tech medical care to basic health care. The shift in goals reflected revised expectations of international equality of health and health provision between people in the developing world and the developed world as health services were expected to orientate themselves around basic needs provision. A primary health care approach, discussed later, was adopted in an international climate more pessimistic about the possibilities and efficacy of progress.

From urban medicine to rural health

Modernisation policies with their emphasis on modern hospitals and medicines encouraged an urban bias in health service spending concentrated on the larger cities. As a consequence, the provision of health care was spread unevenly with more spent on urban areas than rural areas. This urban bias was noted, but was not necessarily condemned. Indeed prioritising provision for urban professionals and industrial workers was deemed an acceptable transitional measure under modernisation approaches as part of fostering a stable nation state and an amenable industrial workforce whose activities were furthering national development for the long-term benefit of the whole population. However, the state national health spending on high-tech hospitals and treatments, which only a tiny percentage of the population had any prospect of accessing, became increasingly criticised as inequitable and wasteful as modernisation approaches themselves were attacked. A 1967 Tanzanian social and policy document, recognising the inequities of the existing health approach, declared:

> We must not forget that people who live in towns can possibly become exploiters of those who live in rural areas. All our big hospitals are in towns and they benefit only a small section of the people of Tanzania; it is the overseas sale of the peasants' produce which provides the foreign exchange of payment. Those who do not get the benefit of the hospitals thus carry the major responsibility for paying for them.[15]

Modern urban hospitals took a large proportion of national health budgets, while public health concerns were not adequately addressed with the over-stretched infrastructure of many cities in developing countries. Housing, sanitation and public services were not keeping pace with the growth of cities, with serious health consequences.

Criticism of the urban bias grew in western official circles along with criticisms of modernisation strategies. Modernisation strategies assumed that urbanisation would lead to urbanism, understood as civic norms of behaviour and values. Instead urban expansion was becoming associated with social problems, epitomised by the vast squatter settlements developing around cities. On the health side, there was alarm that industrial development was not necessarily improving the health of populations, but was spreading disease and creating new health problems. Reports on health in developing countries repeatedly warned against the effects of rapid urbanisation. Urban areas were associated with improved mortality rates, but they were also linked to socially related health problems such as alcoholism, which posed broader concerns for societies. The negative consequences of urbanization for health have been a recurring theme of the last four decades and have been central to sustainable development thinking. In this vein, a collection of essays under the title *Health and Development* published a decade ago cautions that 'urbanization does not automatically equate with better health but it may equate with different health and health problems'.[16]

These social concerns lead back to the WHO's broad definition of health encompassing social well-being and people's capacity to adapt to change. If health is understood as social well-being, then urban social alienation and political unrest imply (in official development thinking) the need to shift away from urbanisation policies.

A negative view of industrialisation and urbanisation is a central theme in the sustainable development literature. The antecedents to sustainable development thinking may be traced back to the Romantic reaction against industrialisation, colonial development policies and anthropological research notably that of the 'Culture and Personality School'. Many anthropologists were preoccupied with the destabilising effects of modernisation on the communities they were observing. Mead's international health study suggested that societies based on tradition were more harmonious and stable:

> People live in accordance with century old-custom, and are emotionally balanced and free from nervous tension because their way of living is closely adapted to the surrounding conditions, into which they were born and in which they will remain all their lives.[17]

Mead's study also suggested the resilience of small-scale traditional rural societies and people's ability to secure their basic needs for food, shelter and health and to adapt to their harsh circumstances.

The negative perceptions of urbanisation led to attacks on the urban bias of international development and a growing preference for rural development to help maintain rural communities and discourage the flight of rural populations to the cities. Sustainable development policies have sought to stabilise communities and promote local solutions, rather than raise people's expectations and encourage social mobility. If sustainable development legitimises different expectations for developing countries than industrialised countries, it does so from a culturally relative perspective, which challenges the earlier development assumptions that developing countries should aspire to become like the advanced industrial societies. An important aspect of this transition was a greater emphasis on primary care.

The primary health care movement

International health policy became centred around the primary health care movement whose ideas were inspired by the evolving sustainable development thinking. Ken Newell, Director of the Division for Strengthening of Health Services at the WHO headquarters from 1971 to 1977, was a key figure. In 1975 Newell's report, *Health by the People,*[18] together with the UNICEF/WHO Study of *Alternative Approaches to Meeting Basic Health Needs of Populations in Developing Countries,*[19] set out the new direction of international health policy. A holistic view of development is reflected in Newell's holistic view of health to include sustaining communities and communal feelings:

> The wider issues presented include: productivity and sufficient resources to enable people to eat and be educated; a sense of community responsibility and involvement; a functioning community organization; self-sufficiency in all important matters and a reliance on outside resources only for emergencies; an understanding of the uniqueness of each community couples with the individual and group pride and dignity associated with it; and lastly, the feeling that people have of a true unity between their land, their work, and their household.[20]

The WHO formally adopted the primary health care approach in 1975. This was followed up by an International Conference on Primary Health Care sponsored by the WHO and UNICEF in 1978. The new international health policy wanted countries to move away from expensive high-tech urban hospital-based curative interventions. Instead of concentrating health services in urban areas, the primary health approach wanted to bring services to people in rural areas. The primary health care movement was influenced by China's use of so called barefoot doctors, non-professional health staff who promoted simple health methods in communities through the workplace and other spaces. Newell described the primary health philosophy as being about more than the delivery of cheap services, and aspiring to move from top-down development and promote grassroots community development giving ordinary people more of a role. Newell summarised its ideals thus:

> Health services were not purely a way of delivering health care interventions to people but were something important to individuals and groups in their own right. Key changes of this idea called primary health care were linked to qualities such as power, ownership, equity and dignity.[21]

The primary health care movement's emphasis on local solutions encouraged the role of non-governmental organisations (NGOs) in community health. Major western relief organisations such as Oxfam reorientated their activities from Europe to developing countries in the post-war period and incorporated development work into their activities. Their needs-based and people-focused relief work has lent itself to sustainable development thinking and they have been well-placed vehicles to carry forward sustainable development ideas. Many NGO staff, like their anthropological predecessors, have partly been inspired to work in the developing world because of their doubts over the character of western industrial societies.

The NGO development philosophy has defined itself against industrial development and embodied local small-scale, technologically simple, community-based development. Their sustainable development philosophy is exemplified in NGO health programmes such as high-profile campaigns against baby-milk formula in favour of breast feeding impassioned by concerns over commercial exploitation by foreign companies. At the same time, public health in NGO development thinking has become attached to environmental concerns where populations in developing countries are constructed as part of nature and protecting their well-being equated with protecting nature. So whereas reference in the older international public health literature to the environment referred to matters such as large-scale public works to improve the infrastructure of cities or clean air legislation, the present reference to the environment is bound up with environmentalist concerns. NGOs, for example, have typically promoted village wells projects and opposed large dam building projects. The links between international health policy and environmental thinking is important in international organisations too, for example, the WHO's Commission on Health and Environment and its report *Our Planet, Our Health*.[22]

Promotion of traditional medicine

The primary health care movement also took a new interest in traditional medicine along with its holistic health approach seeking to respect communities. The changed international health policy involved a shift in the cultural norms considered desirable to foster. If earlier modernisation and health strategies were associated with promoting ambitious risk takers seeking to master nature, the new ideal was associated with enhancing respect for existing cultural identities and harmony with nature. The new interest in traditional medicine reversed the position of earlier international health policy, which saw itself as championing modern scientific medicine against older irrational prejudices, linked to development strategies raising people's horizons beyond their communities.

The 1978 Conference on Primary Health Care and a number of WHO reports including *The Promotion and Development of Traditional Medicine*[23] of the same year endorsed incorporating traditional medicine. The endorsement of traditional medicine was immediately facilitated by the attention given to China's system of primary health and how Chinese health policy integrated both modern and traditional medicine. Receptivity to traditional medicine was encouraged by the inadequate coverage of modern health care services, and further by the revival of interest in traditional medicine among the middle classes in the West and India.[24] The celebration of traditional medicine's integration into primary health care may have romanticised the effective abandonment of universal modern medical health care, but its endorsement was genuine in that it reflected cultural disenchantment with modernity within developed countries and interest in non-industrial cultures as more authentic, ethical ways of life. Traditional medicine compliments notions of sustainable development, appropriate technology and holism. Sustainable development writing characteristically affirms traditional medicine and rejects the idea that traditional medicine is inferior to modern scientifically based medicine. Traditional medicine is generally treated as unproblematic, although occasional concern is voiced that it may impact negatively on the uptake of immunisation programmes.

The next two sections consider radical thinking on international development and health and their contributions to the evolving international health strategies. The first section considers underdevelopment critiques of modernisation and health inequalities. The second section considers counter-culture critiques of modernisation and modern medicine.

Under-development theories and health inequalities

Under-development and dependency theories were the dominant critiques of modernisation in development studies. These influential theories inspired by Marxist and anti-colonial ideas, targeted capitalism and imperialism, rather than industrialisation itself, as perpetuating international inequalities. An under-development theory approach to international health problems is encapsulated in an edited collection of essays entitled *Imperialism, Health and Medicine*.[25] The editor, Vicente Navarro, explains the under-development theory understanding of international health problems:

> The major cause of death and disease in the poor parts of the world today in which the majority of the human race lives is not a scarcity of resources, not the process of industrialization, nor even the much heralded population explosion but, rather, a pattern of control over the resources of those countries in which the majority of the population has no control over their resources.[26]

In summary, his analysis blamed 'the under-development of health' on 'the sickness of imperialism'.[27] Under-development and dependency theories proposed alternative autonomous development models for developing countries outside the world economy dominated by western states, and were interested in the paths of countries such as Cuba, or, Chile under Salvador Allende. The desire to break the dependency of developing countries led under-development critiques to merge with anti-industrialisation critiques. Industrialisation strategies in developing countries were criticised for being reliant on foreign investment and their industrial sectors being subject to foreign domination, ownership and exploitation. Consequently non-industrial economic activities came to be stressed as less dependent. Under-development health thinking sought to break the dependence of developing countries on foreign medical technology and drugs. Under-development thinkers held up Chile's attempt under Allende to move away from national health policies relying on imports of expensive foreign drugs and hospital equipment as exemplary.

Under-development theories were already becoming superseded by anti-industrialisation critiques by the time that the *Imperialism, Health and Medicine* collection of essays was published. The next section discusses the rise of radical anti-industrialisation critiques.

Counter-culture critiques of modern medicine

Official international development thinking became critical of industrialisation as a goal for developing countries and its associated health strategies. Radical international development thinking also adopted anti-industrialisation ideas, although coming from different concerns. Earlier Marxist-inspired accounts had assumed that the industrial proletariat was the agent of social revolution. However, doubts had grown over the political potential of industrial workers following the failures of radical political movements in the late 1960s to bring about fundamental social changes. Counter-culture works such Herbert Marcuse's *One Dimensional Man*[28] or Paulo Freire's *The Pedagogy of the Oppressed*[29] suggested that the hope of radical politics lay with those outside industrial production. A new interest was taken in the role of peasants, particularly following the Vietnamese defeat of the United States in the Vietnam War. Counter-culture ideas mingled with environmental concerns over population growth, resources and the impact of industrialised societies on the planet.

Counter-culture ideas influenced radical thinking on international health. Ivan Illich's works such as *Limits to Medicine, Medical Nemesis*[30] applied anti-modernisation ideas to the health field. Illich, a Catholic priest who lived in Latin America, argued that industrial development was creating frustration, not well-being, and the expansion of wage labour which accompanied industrialisation was undermining autonomy and altruistic relationships.[31] Illich proposed an alternative spiritual view of development and under-development as a state of mind and suggested that domestic or community modes of production as opposed to the wage labour of industrialisation was conducive to altruistic relationships, of relevance to the care of the sick. His work attacked limited health budgets being spent on technologically advanced hospitals and medicines, whose costs were exacerbated by the fact that developing countries had to rely on imports of technology and drugs. He observed that expensive medical training did not necessarily benefit developing countries because trained medical staff could emigrate and find better paid work in developed countries.[32]

Such criticisms echoed criticisms voiced elsewhere. However, Illich's attacks on modernisation and modern medicine were more fundamental. Illich's *Limits to Medicine* proposed that many modern diseases were socially, culturally and professionally constructed, in short, 'man made'.[33] Illich argued for a more holistic concept of health, instead of the modern scientific medical model. Illich wrote of health as freedom, anticipating Amartya Sen's discussion of development as freedom.[34] He was preoccupied with how health intervention smothered 'health-as-freedom' even with equitable provision, although he acknowledged a role for sanitation, inoculation, and vector control. Illich criticised the development of technologically orientated health services for impeding people's self-reliance and therefore undermining people's health – health being defined in terms of autonomy. Furthermore he feared that the development of anaesthetics would anaesthetise people against reality, encouraging passivity and discouraging feelings of compassion:

> An advanced industrial society is sick-making because it disables people from coping with their environment and, when they break down, from substituting a "clinical" prosthesis for the broken relationships. People would rebel against such an environment if medicine did not explain their biological disorientation as a defect in their health, rather than as a defect in the way of life which is imposed on them or which they impose on themselves. The assurance of personal political innocence that a diagnosis offers the patient serves as a hygienic mask that justifies further subjection to production and consumption.[35]

Illich's views may be contrasted with the earlier belief attached to international health policy that medical advances would attack fatalism and raise people's belief in their ability to change their circumstances. Conversely, Illich sees pain as a corrective to humanity's hubris and fears that if humans can be anaesthetised against pain, they will have no sense of limits: 'The pain inflicted on individuals had a limiting effect on the abuses of man by man'.[36] Modern medicine therefore undermined social and moral well-being. Illich's radical rejection of modern medicine was not adopted in international health policy, but his critique of medicalisation helped to legitimise the shift away from the policies aspiring to develop universal modern health services and consolidate the shift to basic health needs for developing countries.

Selective health care strategy

The primary health care ideals of grassroots development were overtaken by economic crisis in the developing world in the 1980s, commonly referred to as a 'lost decade' for development. The imposition of structural adjustment programmes in the wake of the debt crisis in developing countries following the recall of western loans led to serious cutbacks in public services, along with the loss of subsidies on staple foods and the wide imposition of charges, which had implications for the health of populations in the developing world.

NGO activities took on new significance in the 1980s with the international debt crisis and the setbacks in national development. NGOs made trenchant attacks on the impact of structural adjustment programmes on welfare in developing countries and sought ways of limiting their effects. Their debt relief recommendations have sought conditions involving the external regulation of national budgets in developing countries to ensure basic welfare spending including health. Their hopes in external regulation may be contrasted with the earlier dependency theories which were suspicious of outside intervention in developing countries, discussed earlier.

Unsurprisingly the decade witnessed serious reversals in the health gains of the previous decades. Against this backdrop, the primary health care approach was modified into a selective primary health care approach. The selective primary health approach was pioneered by UNICEF and became part of its attempt to facilitate 'adjustment with a human face' and ameliorate the social impact of austerity measures on children. Its GOBI programme identified four simple, cheap and effective health interventions, which could help child survival against the background of the erosion of the already inadequate health services. The programme focused on Growth monitoring, Oral rehydration to counter diarrhoea, Breast feeding and Immunisation against six diseases: tuberculosis, poliomyelitis, diphtheria, tetanus, whooping cough and measles.[37]

The GOBI programme demonstrated real successes in reducing child mortality in an otherwise very depressing decade for international development. Consequently the programme's approach was looked to by other international organisations. The Millennium Development Goals, set out two decades later, are essentially based on UNICEF's approach in the GOBI programme. Indeed Goal Four of the Millennium Development Goals to reduce child mortality incorporates the GOBI programme's strategies with some additions. UNICEF itself expanded the GOBI programme to include 3 Fs: food supplements, family planning, female education.[38] Again this expanded programme had some impact, but the expansion into health education areas of family planning was more controversial and less effective than the original GOBI priorities. The GOBI programme deserves praise for saving lives in the midst of crisis. Good emergency practice is based on the principle of triage, prioritising treatments that save as many lives as possible given insufficient resources in a crisis. However, a selective child survival programme is very far from WHO's objective of 'the attainment by all peoples of the highest possible level of health'. Tellingly primary health care advocates in the 1980s were concerned that a selective health care strategy should not displace a comprehensive primary health care strategy, and criticised its wider adoption as undermining the ideals of the primary health care movement: 'The advocates of highly selected and specific health interventions plus the managerial processes to implement them have ignored, or put on one side, the ideas which are at the core of what could be described as the primary health care revolution. They are in this sense counter revolutionaries'.[39]

These criticisms are interesting given the centrality of the UN Millennium Development Goals in international development planning and campaigning today. If the 1980s were a lost decade for development, and the 1990s were preoccupied with humanitarian work and deprioritised development issues, the new millennium is often presented as re-invigorating development and advancing an exciting innovative and inclusive agenda. Yet the Millennium Development health goals effectively constitute a selective health care strategy. As such the Millennium Development health Goals repackage the 1980s' survival strategies as international development goals. The Millennium Development Goals initiative therefore puts forward a rather demoralised vision for the developing world. So how has present development thinking become reconciled to selective health care strategies?

Voices of the poor

The sustainable development approach has defined itself against the earlier modernisation model based on industrialisation and the trickle-down effect and proposed a bottom-up approach to development. The needs-based approach has evolved into a rights-based approach which has sought to both codify basic needs as a right and to empower the most vulnerable sections of society to realise these rights. So while the earlier sustainable development projects were more focused on practical provision and skills, projects in the last 15 years have become more interested in social empowerment. To name just two influential figures in international development, the economist Amartya Sen has written on *Development as Freedom*,[40] while the aid practitioner John Clark, formerly of Oxfam and more recently adviser to the World Bank has written on *Democratising Development*.[41] The idea of rights-based development has gained acceptance in the World Bank, not just among international social organisations such as the UNDP, WHO and UNICEF.

The empowerment approach to development is encapsulated in the World Bank's seminal *Voices of the Poor* report,[42] officially endorsed by Britain's Department for International Development among other major donors, which has adopted a holistic view of development and sought to take the expressed needs of the poor as the starting point for development work. Thus if the 1980s abandoned primary health care movement concerns over 'power, ownership, equity and dignity',[43] the 1990s saw a revival of interest in these concerns.

The World Bank's *Voices of the Poor* report focuses on individuals at the bottom of society and their personal aspirations, experiences and relationships and sees fulfilment of their modest aspirations as international development priorities. At first glance reorientating development policies around the expressed needs of the poor seems very progressive. Yet international development advisers in the past were concerned with the poor's fatalistic acceptance of their condition and felt they needed to raise populations' expectations. Indeed low expectations are highlighted in the report, which states how its participants 'hope for moderate, not extravagant, improvements'.[44] But orientating policies around people with low expectations leads to minimalist goals. So the report may be accused of disingenuously using the poor's low expectations to legitimise low development goals. The report's authors deny this charge arguing that the importance of small changes identified by the poor reinforces the requirement to prioritise their needs. Yet the empowerment approach has been analysed as legitimising the retreat from state health services and attempting to ensure poor households can improve their own health.[45] The contemporary understanding of well-being also questions the need for significant material transformation to improve the lives and health of populations in developing countries, as the next section discusses. This is another aspect of the *Voices of the Poor* report.

Well-being and the pathologisation of growth

The *Voices of the Poor* report champions the idea that the goal of development should be not wealth but well-being. Its concept of well-being involves 'material well-being, physical well-being, social well-being, security, and freedom of choice and action' contributing to 'states of mind as well as body, in personal psychological experiences of well-being'.[46] Indeed the report suggests that wealth and well-being are not necessarily compatible. Repeatedly the report downplays the significance of material prosperity by highlighting the non-material aspects of well-being.

International development thinking originally emphasised the correlation between a state's wealth, the population's health and health expenditure. But development strategies of the last decade have wanted to counter the idea that a country's wealth necessarily determines the health of the population. Thus the editors of *Health and Development* argued, 'It is by no means clear that health status automatically improves with rising levels of development in any given country, and this certainly cannot be said for all inhabitants'.[47]

The idea underpins the UNDP's annual human development index and reports, which compare the welfare of populations in different countries, highlighting examples where countries with lower national wealth are providing better welfare than those with higher national wealth. The theme is very popular in international development reports today. Favourite examples are Cuba and Kerala province in India. It is often highlighted that Cuba's infant mortality rates compare favourably with the United States of America although Cuba is far less wealthy.

These examples are interesting to study to see if their approaches can be applied elsewhere. Nevertheless a broad correlation remains between a country's wealth and its population's health, although this correlation is downplayed in international development circles today. Sub-Saharan Africa is one of the poorest regions of the world with some of the lowest growth rates and predictably has some of the worst health problems.

Psychological well-being

The elevation of well-being over wealth evidently suggests new possibilities for international health issues to be taken more seriously because the concept of well-being is bound up with health. 'Ill-health is both a cause and a consequence of poverty' is a statement that appears in WHO, World Bank and other international health reports. The World Bank has observed that 'for many poor people, the body is their main asset' and that they 'regard accessible, effective and affordable health treatment as a priority when ranking institutions of local importance'.[48]

The concept of well-being also implies a particular perception of health and health priorities and approaches which is more than the absence of disease. The goal of well-being gives greater emphasis to the psychological aspects of ill-being and well-being, including the psychological aspects of poverty. Unsurprisingly mental health problems have come to the fore. The *Voices of the Poor* report highlighted mental health as a key issue. Mental illness has been made a priority area by the WHO, so too international aid organisations. Indeed the past decade witnessed pointed examples where psychological well-being was prioritised and physical problems downplayed over other health problems in international interventions. Notably the subject of trauma in the 1990s displaced the western media's previous focus on famine as the prism through which developing countries were portrayed. Psychosocial programmes were a core feature of international responses to humanitarian emergencies in the 1990s.[49]

Well-being is bound up with health, but without significant material improvement, populations in developing countries will have to continue to endure many diseases and illnesses that have been eradicated or whose effects are minimised or cured in developed countries through access to modern hospitals and medicines. Yet international development strategies effectively conceptualise the well-being of populations in the developing world as having to accept diseases that fall outside its selective health strategies. As such international development strategies are logically seeking to promote well-being in the presence of disease, not its absence.

Health education strategies

The psychological non-materialist emphasis in international development thinking emphasises solutions at the level of the individual focused primarily on self-help and behaviour modification, rather than the macro level and the eradication of diseases. Health education remains a prime focus of international health policy and is reflected in the recommendations of the World Bank. The report singles out moving from 'illness and incapability to health, information and education',[50] although the report itself acknowledges that the poor emphasise their need for curative medicine. The strategies of the Millennium Goals emphasise education and prevention through behaviour modification rather than cure. *The Millennium Development Goals 2004 Report* on its HIV/AIDs strategy states that 'for the foreseeable future, education will remain the only "vaccine" against HIV' highlighting condom use and behavioural change.[51]

Health education programmes have become the staple response of international aid organisations, but there are questions over the extent of their effectiveness. Health education work has had some success over the decades, but has difficulties achieving universal coverage and universal uptake. Health education programmes tend to overlook the hidden costs of participation in programmes for individuals, such as the burden of time and travel costs to centres. Moreover health education work (including Millennium Development Goals initiatives) often confuses problems of knowledge, acceptance and behaviour changes. Research on the effectiveness of health education has long highlighted the importance of distinguishing knowledge, attitudes and behaviour change. Even if people are informed about risks, there may be difficulty persuading people to follow precautionary health messages when people's lives are inherently insecure. Communities may have developed traditional risk avoidance strategies following traditional patterns. However, there are few incentives to adopt new patterns of behaviour based on modern risk avoidance if one does not expect one's life to be significantly transformed. Mead's study on *Culture, Health and Disease* 40 years ago understood this problem,[52] yet such experience is repeatedly overlooked.

Contrasting visions of global health

The new emphasis on global health draws attention to how health threats transcend borders, but these borders remain as relevant today as before in determining the health of populations. Too often disproportionate attention in global health is given to potential risks posed by diseases in the developing countries to western countries as opposed to the daily experience of disease and ill health in developing countries. Moreover some of the diseases such as ebola that have received much publicity as global health threats in recent years appear to reflect irrational panics rather than realistic threats. So while international development policies emphasise the problem of inequalities, the emphasis is on inequalities within developing countries, between rural and urban, gender inequalities within families, but have surprisingly little to say on international inequalities nor do they express an aspiration for developing countries to have the same standard of health as those in developed countries.

International health advocacy, for all the reference to being part of a global village, has not challenged the unspoken assumption of international health inequalities, that populations in developing countries cannot expect to have modern health systems based on the latest medical developments. The well-being of populations in developing countries, it seems, is to be based on their stoical acceptance of a materially simple life. The empowerment of the poor does not encompass adoption of the same standards of living and expectations of populations in developed countries. Indicatively participants in a workshop on human rights led by British lawyers in Bosnia were instructed that the right to health concerned the right to basic health, not advanced cancer treatment.

Recently there has been more international advocacy around patenting and the availability of cheap generic medicines taken up by NGOs such as MSF and Oxfam. Again the problem of developing countries losing health workers to western health systems, for example, is currently receiving concern. Renewed attention is also being given to the major diseases of malaria and tuberculosis. However, international advocacy remains informed by different development and health expectations for developing countries. Although these differences are based on cultural relativist arguments, rather than elitist arguments, they are nevertheless legitimising unequal health outcomes.

Exceptionally the Bill and Melinda Gates Foundation, founded by the billionaire Microsoft entrepreneur Bill Gates, states an aspiration for health expectation in developing countries to be the same as that in the West: 'The mission of our Global Health program is to ensure that people in the developing world have the same chance for good health as people in the developed world'.[53]

Strikingly this aspiration for equality in health between developing and developed countries has come from an organisation outside of international development circles which have inculcated low expectations. The high aspirations for health in developing countries represent a breath of fresh air, shaking up international health debates, and are also backed by real resources, which however small relative to the problems, might result in some scientific breakthroughs that could help cure and eradicate diseases and inspire more official action. The audacity of the ideas invokes the earlier spirit of international health planning. The announcement of Gates that his foundation was going to put resources into seeking a cure for malaria and a method of eradicating malaria-carrying mosquitoes resurrect some of the ambitions around the MEP of half a century ago. International NGOs have welcomed the new initiatives, but there is some ambivalence. In key respects, Gates's approach is antithetical to contemporary international development and international health thinking. Notably research into developing disease resistant crops with enhanced nutrients involving genetic modification, or genetically modifying mosquitoes to eradicate malaria-carrying mosquitoes, or developing new insecticides goes against sustainable development thinking. Such ambitions invoke the spectre of humanity's hubris, which has haunted development thinking for the last three decades.

Conclusion

The presence of disease and sickness is the reality for populations in developing countries. Most of the world's population remain without access to both adequate primary health care and medically advanced interventions. The vast majority of health problems suffered by people in developing countries are unaddressed. With few exceptions, the 'attainment by all peoples of the highest possible level of health'[54] does not appear to be an objective any longer, let alone a reality.

Discussion topics

- How might the shift in international health policy away from 'modernisation' towards 'sustainable development' affect the health of people in the third world?
- Are the changes in international health policy a realistic response to the social and economic conditions prevailing in the third world, or, do they reflect a broader crisis in the western medical model?
- Compare and contrast the health problems of the United Kingdom with those of sub-Saharan Africa; to what extent do they require similar solutions?

Further reading

Mead, M. (1966) *Culture, Health and Disease: Social and Cultural Influence on Health Programmes in Developing Countries*. London: Tavistock.

Narayan, D., Chambers, R., Kaul Shah, M. and Petesch, P. (eds) (2000) *Voices of the Poor: Crying Out for Change*. Oxford: Oxford University Press for the World Bank.

Navarro, Vicente (ed.) (1982) *Imperialism, Health and Medicine*. London: Pluto.

Pupavac, Vanessa (2006) Humanitarian politics and the rise of international disaster psychology. In Gilbert Reyes and Gerald Jacobs (eds), *Handbook of International Disaster Psychology*. Westport, CT: Praeger.

References

1 World Health Organisation (1948) *Constitution*. Available at http://www. who.int
2 Cowen, M. and Shenton, R. (1995) The invention of development. In J. Crush (ed.), *The Power of Development*. London: Routledge.

3   Furedi, F. (1997) *Population and Development*. Cambridge: Polity.
4   Sorkin, A.L. (1976) *Health Economics in Developing Countries*. Lexington, MA: Lexington Books, p. 120.
5   Malenbaum, W.L. (1970) Health and productivity in poor areas. In H. Klarman (ed.), *Empirical Statistics in Health Economies*. Baltimore, MD: Johns Hopkins Press.
6   Mead, M. (1966) *Culture, Health and Disease: Social and Cultural Influence on Health Programmes in Developing Countries*. London: Tavistock, p. 86.
7   Mead, M. (1966),ibid. p. 89.
8   Carson, R. (1965) *Silent Spring*. London: Penguin.
9   Seers, D. (1979) The meaning of development. In D. Lehmann (ed.), *Development Theory: Four Critical Studies*. London: Frank Cass, p. 9.
10 Brandt Report (1980) Independent Commission on International Development Issues (1980) *North–South: A Programme for Survival*. London: Pan Books, p. 24.
11 ILO (1969) *The World Employment Programme. Report of the Director General of the ILO (part 1) to the International Labour Conference*. Geneva: ILO.
12 ILO (1976) *Employment Growth and Basic Needs: One World Problem. Report of the Director General of the ILO*. Geneva: ILO.
13 Seers, D. (1979) ibid.
14 Schumacher, E.F. (1973) *Small Is Beautiful: A Study of Economics as if People Mattered*. London: Blond & Briggs.
15 Arusha Declaration, quoted by Chagula, W.K. and Tarimo, E. (1975) Meeting basic health needs in Tanzania. In Ken Newell (ed.), *Health by the People*. Geneva: WHO, p. 151.
16 Phillips, D. and Verhasselt, Y. (eds) (1994) *Health and Development*. London: Routledge, p. 151.
17 Mead, M. (1966) ibid., p. 4.
18 Newell, K. (ed.) (1975) *Health by the People*. Geneva: WHO.
19 Djukanovic, V. and Mach, E.P. (eds) (1975) *Alternative Approaches to Meeting Basic Health Needs of Populations in Developing Countries: A Joint UNICEF/WHO Study*. Geneva: WHO.
20 Newell, K. (ed.) ibid., p. 192.
21 Newell, K. (1988) Selective primary health care: the counter revolution. *Social Science and Medicine*, 26: 903–6.
22 WHO (1992) *Our Planet, Our Health: Report of the WHO Commission on Health and the Environment*. Geneva: WHO.
23 WHO (1978) *The Promotion and Development of Traditional Medicine*. Geneva: WHO.
24 Leslie, C. (ed.) (1976) *Asian Medical Systems: A Comparative Study*. London: University of California Press.
25 Navarro, V. (ed.) (1982) *Imperialism, Health and Medicine*. London: Pluto.
26 Navarro, V. (ed.) (1982) ibid., p. 7.
27 Navarro, V. (ed.) ibid., p. 9.
28 Marcuse, H. (1964) *One Dimensional Man: Studies in the Ideology of Advanced Industrial Society*. Boston, MA: Beacon Press.
29 Freire, P. (1972) *The Pedagogy of the Oppressed*. Harmondsworth: Penguin.
30 Illich, I. (1976) *Limits to Medicine, Medical Nemesis: The Expropriation of Health*. London: Marion Boyars.
31 Illich, I. (1976) ibid., pp. 215–16.
32 Illich, I. (1976) ibid., p. 56.

33 Illich, I. (1976) ibid., p. 107.
34 Sen, A. (1999) *Development as Freedom*. Oxford: Oxford University Press.
35 Illich, I. (1976) ibid., p. 169.
36 Illich, I. (1976) ibid., p. 135.
37 Black, M. (1996) *Children First: The Story of UNICEF, Past and Present*. Oxford: Oxford University Press, pp. 18–19.
38 Black, M. (1996) ibid.
39 Newell, K. (1988) ibid.
40 Sen, A. (1999) ibid.
41 Clark, J. (1992) Democratising development: NGOs and the state. *Development in Practice*, 2(3): 151–62.
42 Narayan, D., Chambers, R., Kaul Shah, M. and Petesch, P. (eds) (2000) *Voices of the Poor: Crying Out for Change*. Oxford: Oxford University Press for the World Bank.
43 Newell, K. (1988) ibid.
44 Narayan, D., Chambers, R., Kaul Shah, M. and Petesch, P. (eds) (2000) ibid., p. 24.
45 Abrahamsen, R. (2000) *Disciplining Democracy: Development Discourse and Good Governance in Africa*. London: Zed Books.
46 Narayan, D., Chambers, R., Kaul Shah, M. and Petesch, P. (eds) (2000) ibid., p. 22.
47 Phillips, D. and Verhasselt, Y. (eds) (1994) *Health and Development*. London: Routledge, p. xiv.
48 Narayan, D., Chambers, R., Kaul Shah, M. and Petesch, P. (eds) (2000) ibid., p. 100.
49 Pupavac, V. (2006) Humanitarian politics and the rise of international disaster psychology. In Gilbert Reyes and Gerald Jacobs (eds), *Handbook of International Disaster Psychology*. Westport, CT: Praeger, pp. 15–34.
50 Narayan, D., Chambers, R., Kaul Shah, M. and Petesch, P. (eds) (2000) ibid., p. 263.
51 United Nations (2004) *Millennium Development Goals 2004 Report*. Available at http://www.un.org/millenniumgoals/
52 Mead, M. (1966) *Culture, Health and Disease: Social and Cultural Influence on Health Programmes in Developing Countries*. London: Tavistock.
53 Bill and Melinda Gates Foundation website http://www.gatesfoundation.org
54 World Health Organisation (1948) *Constitution*. Available at http://www.who.int

Conclusion

> Finally ... some remarks are in order about how – or, indeed, whether – the practice of sociology would need to be different in my 're-imagined' form. Certainly the word 'sociology' would recover its original normative voice, as disciplinary practitioners see themselves contributing to the constitution of the societies they study, typically by raising subjects' collective self-consciousness.
>
> Steve Fuller, *The New Sociological Imagination*, 2006

This book has spanned a broad terrain, from the putative health risks of mobile phones to the government's 'expert patient programme', and from the growing popularity of homeopathy to the construction of new maladies, such as fibromyalgia or work stress. Superficially, these phenomena appear to be independent and discrete, however, closer analysis reveals common threads, which when drawn together help us to understand what is unique and historically specific about the prevailing discourse of health.

The unifying theme and the key to understanding contemporary health issues is the concept of *fear*. Fear is manifest at two interlinked levels of analysis, at the individual and the social, or to use C.Wright Mills's terminology, personal troubles and public issues.[1] At both levels of analysis there are two aspects to this new wave of anxiety. First, is a heightened sense of vulnerability to mental and physical pathology and to the unchecked power of vested interests. The second aspect is a diminished sense of agency; the belief that we are largely powerless to overcome these external threats.

The heightened sense of vulnerability can be seen in the epidemic of 'health scares' which suggests that previously taken-for-granted aspects of everyday life, such as, diet, paid employment, or the use of new technologies, pose a major threat to our physical or mental health. The list of perceived threats extends to institutionalised structures of power which were previously thought to be benign or even beneficent. The pharmaceutical industry, whose products have saved countless lives, is derided as 'Big Pharma' and the medical profession itself is constantly disparaged as a source of abuse, by reference to high profile 'scandals' such as the postmortem removal and retention (without parental consent) of children's organs by pathologists at the Alder Hay Hospital, or the furore around expert witness Professor Roy Meadows's erroneous evidence, which contributed to the wrongful conviction of several women accused of murdering their children. The point is not that such threats are false, or that they do not warrant investigation, but that their magnitude is grossly amplified; the personal and institutional responses they evoke are disproportionate to the actual threat posed; and that this over-reaction can generate adverse outcomes which outweigh those of the perceived threat.

The individual and social responses to these perceived threats illustrate the second aspect of the contemporary form of fear, namely the diminished sense of agency or selfhood. Superficially, it appears contradictory to insist that examples of individual and social action illustrate a diminution of agency. However, by agency, we are not referring to any and all forms of activity, but to purposive human action to transform and humanise the external world. Thus when the Inquisition arrested Galileo and branded his support for heliocentrism heretical, they were not engaging in human agency, but trying to stifle it. The response to the contemporary culture of fear is equally conservative and counter to human agency. At both the individual and collective levels the response is characterised by the *precautionary principle* which holds that no action should be taken unless its consequences can be proven to be benign.

As we have seen, at the institutional level this has led to new forms of regulation, which have placed constraints on scientific development and reduced the autonomy of the medical profession. At the individual level, the diminished sense of agency has generated an introspective and internalised response, characterised by risk avoidance and the tendency to translate social problems into medical complaints, giving rise to a host of new syndromes. Rather than trying to change the world, individuals attempt to resolve their problems by seeking therapeutic solutions or by calling for ever greater regulation of health risks and unhealthy lifestyles.

Another aspect of the response to the culture of fear is the promotion of *faux democracy*, this impulse relates not so much to the political sphere as to professional and scientific hierarchies. It goes beyond the imposition of regulatory mechanisms, to challenge the authority of scientific knowledge and professional expertise, which are often dismissed as elitist or undemocratic. The notion of *medical pluralism* encapsulates this perspective, implying that clinical science is merely one voice which should possess no greater authority than that of the 'expert patient' or the alternative therapist. While this approach appears egalitarian it is essentially an entirely false form of democracy, as it runs counter to the production of rational discourse on which genuinely democratic decision making is based. It is also profoundly agency robbing, as it undermines the role of reason in transforming the natural and social world, in favour of partial knowledge and superstition.[2] This retreat from reason marks a significant lowering of expectations regarding the capacity for human agency to transform the world we live in, which as we have seen is particularly bleak when applied to the process of Third World development.

Taken together, the heightened sense of vulnerability and the diminished sense of agency reveal what is new and unique about the prevailing culture of fear. Other cultures *really were* vulnerable to external threats, the plague reduced the population of Europe by at least a third in the fourteenth century, and more recently up to 1 million people died in the Irish Potato famine of the late 1840s. The peasants of medieval Europe *really were* powerless to resist the spread of infectious disease, and in the mid-nineteenth century the Irish *really were* unable to overcome the food shortages caused by potato blight and English colonialism. Contemporary developed societies are not free from objective threats to health, but what is unique about the prevailing culture of fear is the mis-match between the magnitude of the threat on one hand, and on the other our heightened sense of perceived vulnerability and diminished sense of capacity to overcome these threats.

It is in this context that the new discourse of health should be understood. Its central characteristics are both a product of and contributor to a broader anti-humanist current. Popular culture often asserts that humanity needs to 'reduce its footprint on the Earth', to intervene less in nature. The growing human population is frequently represented as a form of global disease that is stifling the planet. The achievements of modern medicine in extending life expectancy are often presented as part of this 'problem'.

Medical sociology has in some instances contributed to this anti-humanist world-view, however, it also has an important role to play in de-bunking it. The new discourse of health is very different to that of thirty years ago. Although new technologies and medical advances continue to emerge, they are often received with ambivalence and suspicion. The Enlightenment project of using science and reason to create 'heaven on Earth' is frequently dismissed as hubristic. There is a new culture of fear, vulnerability and uncertainty that threatens to undermine medical progress. These changes have sociological origins, and it is only by exploring those origins and bringing them into public consciousness that the prevailing anti-humanism can be challenged.

References

1 Mills, C.W. (1959) *The Sociological Imagination*. New York: Oxford University Press.
2 Taverne, D. (2006) *The March of Unreason: Science, Democracy and the New Fundamentalism*. Oxford: Oxford University Press.

Index